FRAILTY FIGHTERS

Steps to a Healthier Aging

Dr Saifuddin Ekram

Independently Published

ISBN: 9798304074438
Independently Published

Cover design by: Art Painter

Printed in the United States of America

In loving memory of my parents. You are my forever inspiration.

CONTENTS

Title Page

Copyright

Dedication

Introduction

Chapter 1: Why Frailty Matters 1

Chapter 2: What Frailty Means 9

Chapter 3: The Power of Muscles 16

Chapter 4: Bone Health 23

Chapter 5: Mind-Body Connection 31

Chapter 6: Flexibility for Life 39

Chapter 7: The Fuel Factor 47

Chapter 8: Role of Sleep 56

Chapter 9: Heart Health and Beyond 64

Chapter 10: Stress Busters 72

Chapter 11: Role of Balance 78

Chapter 12: Social Health 86

Chapter 13: Building Resilience 94

Chapter 14: Long-Term Plan 101

Chapter 15: Blueprint for a Frailty-Free Future 109

Abbreviations 118

References 119

Books By This Author 123

Aging Journey

Aging is a journey we all embark upon, but how we navigate it makes all the difference. For some, the golden years are a time of vitality and purpose. For others, they bring challenges, limitations, and a sense of decline. The difference often comes down to one critical factor: frailty—or rather, the ability to prevent it.

Frailty is not just about weakness or vulnerability; it's a complex interplay of physical, mental, and emotional health that can profoundly affect our quality of life. Yet, it is not an inevitable outcome of aging. In fact, science increasingly shows that with the right lifestyle choices, we can delay, mitigate, or even reverse frailty. The goal of this book is to empower you with the knowledge, tools, and inspiration to do just that.

Why This Book Matters

'Frailty Fighters' is your comprehensive guide to understanding and tackling frailty from every angle. It's not just about avoiding decline; it's about thriving—building strength, resilience, and joy at every stage of life. Whether you're in your 40s, 60s, or beyond, this book offers actionable steps to help you take charge of your health and future.

As you turn these pages, you'll find simple explanations of complex topics, practical advice grounded in science, and a blueprint for living stronger, healthier, and more connected. You'll learn about the power of muscles, the importance of nutrition, the role of sleep, and the value of social connections. You'll discover how to set goals, celebrate progress, and create a long-term plan that works for you.

What Makes This Book Unique

Unlike books that focus solely on one aspect of aging, 'Frailty Fighters' offers a holistic approach. It connects the dots between physical strength, cognitive health, emotional resilience, and social well-being. It's not about quick fixes or impossible routines; it's about realistic, sustainable changes that fit into your life, no matter what your starting point.

Most importantly, this book isn't just about information—it's about transformation. It's a call to action, a source of encouragement, and a roadmap to a healthier, happier future.

A Shared Vision

Imagine a world where aging doesn't mean slowing down or stepping back but instead becoming stronger, wiser, and more capable. This vision isn't just aspirational; it's achievable. It starts with understanding frailty and taking the steps to prevent it. And it starts with you. As you embark on this journey, remember that every small choice you make today contributes to a brighter, more resilient tomorrow. Let this book be your guide, your companion, and your cheerleader as you take the steps to fight frailty and embrace healthier aging.

Welcome to a journey of strength, vitality, and lifelong resilience. Welcome to 'Frailty Fighters: Steps to a Healthier Aging'.

Frailty—What Is It, And Why Start Preventing It Now?

When you hear "frailty," you might picture someone shuffling with a walker or squinting at a pillbox. And while that's a part of the story, there's way more to it than meets the eye. Frailty isn't just about old age; it's a condition grounded in science, measured with tools like Fried Frailty Phenotype (FFP) (1) and the Frailty Index (FI) (2). These standardized measures help doctors and researchers define frailty, whether it's a gradual accumulation of deficits over time or specific symptoms like weakness and exhaustion. Think of them as the yardsticks that help us track and tackle frailty more effectively.

So, what exactly is frailty? Picture it as your body's ability to roll with the punches slowly wearing thin. It's not just about having a bad day; it's when small stressors—like a cold or climbing stairs—start feeling like full-blown battles. Frailty is a medical condition that reduces physical resilience and strength, making it tougher to recover from life's curveballs (3). Standardized measures like the FFP or FI have shown us that frailty isn't one-size-fits-all; it's a spectrum influenced by everything from genetics to lifestyle choices and even your socio-economic environment (4).

It is clear that frailty is a complex condition, and there are various ways to classify it, but no single method has emerged as the gold standard (5). Here's an overview of the key approaches:

Physical Frailty: This is the most common way to classify frailty and is often based on the "frailty phenotype," which focuses on five key symptoms: unintentional weight loss, weakness, slow walking speed, low physical activity, and exhaustion. If you meet three or more of these, you're considered frail.

Deficit Accumulation: This method, also known as the "frailty index," looks at the presence of multiple health problems or deficits—such as chronic conditions, disabilities, or poor cognition. The more deficits you have, the more frail you are. It's a broader and more flexible approach, but it requires a lot of data.

Comprehensive Geriatric Assessment (CGA): This holistic approach includes evaluating not only physical health but also cognitive and social well-being. CGA is used in clinical settings to understand an individual's overall health, but it's resource-intensive and not always feasible outside of medical facilities.

Clinical Frailty Scale (CFS): This scale provides a simple rating system from 1 (very fit) to 9 (terminally ill). It's widely used in clinical practice for its simplicity and ease of application, but it doesn't always capture the subtleties of frailty, like physical function or the psychological aspect.

Multidimensional Frailty: Some models combine elements of physical frailty, cognitive decline, and other factors (like nutrition and mental health) into one comprehensive classification. These are useful for research but are more complex to implement.

No classification method stands alone as the definitive measure of frailty. Each approach has strengths and weaknesses, depending on the context—whether it's clinical practice, research, or population health studies (5). The variety of methods reflects the complexity of frailty itself.

Now, here's where the plot thickens: while frailty has roots in factors you can't always control (thanks, genetics), it's also shaped by what you do every day. Frailty often results from a combination of biological aging processes and environmental factors that can weaken the body over time. The mechanisms behind frailty involve declines in muscle mass and strength, reduced physical activity, and imbalances in the body's hormonal and immune systems, which can lead to greater vulnerability to illness and disability. Yes, lifestyle tweaks—like moving more, eating better, and sleeping well—can make a difference by helping to preserve muscle and cognitive function, and by reducing inflammation. But let's not kid ourselves; no amount of kale smoothies can entirely override a lifetime of challenges like poverty, chronic stress, or limited access to healthcare. The goal isn't perfection but progress—stacking the odds in your favor wherever you can.

Think of preventing frailty like planning for retirement. You wouldn't wait until your bank account is empty to start saving, right? Just as financial advisors harp on about compound interest, your body benefits from early investments too. Choices made in your 20s, 30s, and 40s—from staying active to managing stress—build what researchers call your "resilience reserve." This is your safety net for the decades to come, and trust me, future-you will thank present-you for it. And let's not forget the social side of frailty. It's not just about biology; it's about community and connection. Studies show that people with strong social ties tend to age better (6)—so call your friends, join that book club, or take up pickleball. Frailty prevention isn't just a solo gig; it's a team sport.

The takeaway? Frailty isn't inevitable, but it's also not entirely avoidable. It's a mix of nature, nurture, and effort—with a sprinkle of good luck.

Frailty Isn't Just for Grandparents—It's a Slow Build Over Decades

Frailty often carries a stigma as something that only affects the old, but in reality, it's a slow-built condition that starts far sooner than most realize. True, frailty in older adults may come with outward signs—slower movement, reduced strength, and overall fatigue—but it's not something that appears overnight. It develops gradually, starting quietly and subtly in younger years. Imagine it like a hidden app draining your phone battery: you're going about your day, not noticing that somewhere quietly, a little bit of energy is slipping away.

What's more, frailty doesn't just mean physical weakness. It's a cocktail of decreased strength, lower energy, and reduced resilience that touches every aspect of health, including mental well-being and social engagement. So, if your lifestyle now includes regular slouching, sleep deprivation, or a steady diet of processed foods, consider that these habits might be setting you up for a weaker foundation in the long run. Fortunately, while frailty can creep in slowly, it's also a process we have considerable control over, especially if we start early (7).

Why Frailty Prevention Starts Now: Investing in Resilience for Life

Picture yourself in your 20s: you're pulling all-nighters, dancing till dawn, or hauling grocery bags without a second thought. Right now, you may feel invincible, but those invincibility days don't last forever. Here's the kicker: even while you're enjoying the peak energy of youth, habits are setting the stage for how your body and mind will age. While some aspects of aging are beyond our control, research shows that healthy habits, built over time, lay a strong foundation for resilience against frailty.

Think of it as a health savings account: every balanced meal, every workout, every good night's sleep is a deposit that your future self can withdraw from. Skimp on these "deposits" now, and you may find yourself with an empty account when you need it most. Imagine that each walk, each stretch, and every bit of strength training today is like storing strength and vitality for future decades. It's less about preventing frailty outright and more about equipping yourself with the tools to handle whatever comes your way, at any age.

The Slow, Stealthy Path of Frailty: A Cautionary Tale

Frailty is a quiet issue; it doesn't rush in with alarms or warnings. In our younger years, we rarely think about muscle strength or bone density, assuming that these things will always "be there." Yet, studies show that many frailty indicators can begin to accumulate decades before we see any outward signs (8). Think of frailty as a hidden app running in the background, chipping away at your physical and mental resilience while you're preoccupied with everyday life. But unlike other apps, this one doesn't have an "off" button. Instead, it requires intentional effort to slow it down.

In practical terms, what does this look like? Start by visualizing what life looks like down the road. Small choices, like taking the stairs, staying active, and making time for healthy meals, are more than feel-good tips; they're the building blocks of resilience. It's about giving your body what it needs to thrive in the years to come, little by little, so that "older you" won't struggle with what "younger you" took for granted.

Why We're All a Little Frail Already (Yes, really!)

Here's a reality check: moments of frailty aren't exclusive to older adults. Ever felt sore for days after an intense workout? Or like your couch became a part of you after a Netflix binge? Those glimpses of stiffness and sluggish recovery are like mini previews of frailty, moments when your youthful resilience dips. These temporary aches and slumps may seem harmless now, but the fact is, recovery times naturally slow as we age. So, while you may bounce back from a hard workout now, that same recovery will take longer in a few decades.

This doesn't mean you should avoid challenging yourself, but rather that supporting your body with rest, strength training, and nutritious fuel matters more than we tend to think. Look at it like strength training for your future self. Today's balanced meals, regular movement, and full nights of sleep are the physical and mental "armor" that will serve you down the road.

Building Your Frailty Insurance: It's Easier Than You Think!

Think of building frailty resilience as your "frailty insurance policy." There are no premiums to pay and no lengthy paperwork; it's just a few straightforward habits that keep you active, strong, and resilient over time. Preventing frailty doesn't mean cutting out the good things in life; it's about small, achievable habits that add up. Start by walking a little more, adding veggies to your meals, doing some strength exercises, and getting restful sleep. Your body is like a dynamic, adaptable machine. Treat it with respect, and it will serve you well in the long run. Sure, it's easy to think, "I'll worry about frailty when I'm older." But here's a truth few realize: "later" sneaks up faster than we think. The choices you make today help ensure that in the future-you is active, agile, and resilient. A little effort now can mean decades of health and vitality ahead. So, embrace this "frailty-free" journey now—it's the best gift you can give yourself.

Aging, Resilience, And The Whole Package—Physical, Mental, And Social Health

Aging is like an extreme sport where everyone's invited, whether they're ready or not! Picture it this way: frailty prevention is a marathon, but not the kind where you're chugging energy drinks and hoping to make it to the finish line. This is a whole-body workout that calls for a blend of strength, resilience, and a sense of humour—after all, laughter really is the best medicine. Frailty prevention isn't just about maintaining physical health; it's about cultivating resilience across all facets of life: physical, mental, and social (9). Each of these elements acts as a pillar holding up the temple of your health, and when one starts to falter, the others can feel it too. So, if you think about it, you're not just an assortment of cells, muscles, and bones; you're an interconnected ecosystem.

Physical Health: Keeping the Body Agile

Physically, aging doesn't mean you're doomed to a life of aching joints and endless couch time. While it's true that aging cells repair more slowly, the body remains remarkably adaptable, even in later years. Let's start with the muscles: yes, they might lose a bit of their former bulk, but with regular activity, they can stay strong and even grow! Think of muscle as the body's secret anti-aging elixir. A consistent routine of resistance exercises or weight training can help you keep up your strength, making things like climbing stairs or lifting groceries seem like mere warm-ups.

Bones might seem a bit trickier. With age, bones tend to lose density, especially after 30, when bone resorption can outpace formation. But the good news? Weight-bearing exercises—like jogging, dancing, and stair climbing—send little shocks through your bones, which encourage them to stay strong (10). And it's not just for your bones; your heart and lungs will thank you too. Regular aerobic exercise boosts circulation, which doesn't just help prevent frailty but also makes you feel more energized (11). Think of your daily walk as a "multi-vitamin" for your whole body—each step strengthens not only muscles and bones but even your mental health.

Speaking of your brain, let's not overlook the enormous benefits exercise provides for your mind. Physical activity has been shown to reduce stress, elevate mood, and even slow cognitive decline. So, when you're walking or lifting those dumbbells, you're doing a bit of brain training too. This keeps you sharp, motivated, and ready for whatever challenges come your way—because, as we'll see, resilience isn't just a physical trait.

Mental Health: Flexing the Mind

Just as muscles need a bit of stress to stay strong, so does the mind. Our brains crave stimulation, especially as we age. Frailty isn't only a physical state; it's also a mindset. A positive outlook on aging—seeing it not as a decline but as a phase rich with opportunity—can have profound effects on how we age. People with this mindset are more likely to stay physically active, socially engaged, and even live longer. A bit of optimism acts like a natural painkiller, helping to buffer against the everyday stresses that come with getting older.

Mental health, in this context, is like a dynamic workout for the brain. Tackling puzzles, learning new things, reading, or even diving into creative projects—these activities are like squats and lunges for the mind, strengthening mental resilience bit by bit. Studies show that people who stay mentally active and participation in leisure activities have a lower risk of dementia and cognitive decline (12). But it's not just about crossword puzzles and sudoku. Purpose is a potent force in mental health. Having goals, even small ones, gives a sense of direction and achievement. This doesn't have to be a monumental undertaking—taking up gardening, starting a book club, or volunteering can provide that same sense of purpose and direction.

In short, nurturing mental health is like installing a backup system for your resilience. When we remain engaged and motivated, it's easier to take on life's little (and big) challenges. Mental toughness supports physical endurance, and, as we'll see, it's also a major player in social health.

Social Health: The Glue Holding It All Together

Of all the pillars of resilience, social health is perhaps the most underrated. Humans are wired to connect, and meaningful relationships can be just as crucial to health as any diet or exercise routine. Studies reveal that social isolation can lead to numerous health problems, including heart disease, depression, and—you guessed it—frailty (6, 13). Social connections provide not only companionship but also accountability. Having a friend to go on walks with, someone to chat with over tea, or just knowing your part of a larger community can motivate you to stay active and mentally engaged.

Social health isn't just about avoiding loneliness; it's a powerhouse of mental and physical benefits. Engaging with others stimulates the brain, often in more complex ways than solo activities. Think of a casual conversation over coffee—your brain is processing facial expressions, recalling details, responding to cues, and engaging in real-time problem-solving. These are mini mental workouts that keep your mind sharp. And on a physical level, social interactions can even boost immune function, reducing inflammation and the risks associated with aging.

Even better? Social health fosters resilience in ways that aren't always obvious. When life throws a curveball, it's often friends and family who help us bounce back. This is why building and nurturing relationships can be seen as "frailty insurance." In a society that sometimes prizes independence to a fault, embracing the idea that it's okay to rely on others can be transformative.

Synergy in Action: The Interplay of Physical, Mental, and Social Health

Imagine each of these health aspects—physical, mental, and social—as legs of a stool. If one leg wobbles, the whole structure becomes unstable. This interconnection is the core of resilience. Physical health gives you the strength to participate in social activities and fuels mental sharpness. Mental health keeps you motivated to exercise and engage with others. And social health provides emotional support to maintain physical routines and bounce back from setbacks. Each leg strengthens the others, creating a sturdy foundation against frailty.

Consider an example: a retiree who joins a dance class. Physically, they're getting a workout that benefits their muscles, bones, and heart. Mentally, they're challenged to learn new moves and follow rhythm, which keeps their brain active and engaged. Socially, they're connecting with others, building friendships, and sharing laughter, all of which boost mood and reduce stress. Together, these activities weave a strong net of resilience, protecting against the creep of frailty.

The Frailty-Free Package: Embracing the Whole Package

The path to healthy aging isn't about focusing on just one area. It's about embracing all aspects of health to create a life that's not only long but rich in vitality. Physical strength allows for mental agility, mental agility supports social engagement, and social engagement enhances physical and mental resilience. Aging, then, becomes less of a slow decline and more of a graceful evolution.

Preventing frailty means taking small, consistent steps that support your body, mind, and social life. Physical activity, mental engagement, and social connection aren't just "nice to haves"; they're essential, each a vital piece of the puzzle. So, as you age, think of yourself as a complex ecosystem, a whole package that thrives when every part of you is nourished. Embrace this whole- body sport of aging with a light heart, and remember: every walk, every laugh, every puzzle solved is building the foundation for a resilient, frailty-free future.

Everyday Habits That Sneakily Contribute To Frailty

Alright, let's dig deeper into these everyday habits that seem innocent but can eventually knock on the door of frailty. They may look small, but over time, they pile up to be as noticeable as that junk drawer you've been ignoring! Let's look at how everyday choices have lasting effects, one small decision at a time.

Okay, so we've established that frailty is a full-body issue—connected to physical, mental, and social resilience. But what's behind it? The answer might surprise you: it's our everyday habits. Yes, the little choices we make (or avoid) daily are the culprits! Picture it like this: each "I'll skip the gym today" or "just one more episode" moment is a sneaky little jinx, chipping away at our future vitality. Let's look at some classic offenders.

Sitting Too Much: The "Office Chair Olympics"

If sitting was a competitive sport, we'd all be champions. Between work, commuting, meals, and unwinding, it's shocking how much of our day is spent parked in a chair. And let's face it—our bodies weren't designed to lounge around all day! All that sitting isn't just a recipe for stiffness; it shortens muscles, messes with our posture, and weakens the same muscles we need to stay mobile and balanced.

Now, some people might think, "But I'm resting!" While rest is essential, prolonged inactivity is like putting your muscles on "hibernate mode." It's the sneakiest path to frailty, especially as those vital muscles we use for walking, bending, and balancing get weaker. To combat this, sprinkle a little activity into your day. Try setting an alarm to stand, stretch, or take a lap every hour. Desk stretches, mini yoga moves, or even calf raises while waiting for the kettle can do wonders to keep your body awake and engaged.

The Great Diet Conundrum: "But It Was Only One Slice of Pizza!"

Diet plays an enormous role in how we age, yet for many, healthy eating feels like it's "optional." It's easy to see why; eating a salad isn't as satisfying as a burger in the short term. But here's the thing: the fuel you put into your body determines your energy levels, bone density, muscle function, and even brainpower over time.

When the usual menu leans toward pizza, fries, and sugary treats, it doesn't take long for our bones and muscles to start running on empty. Those processed foods may fill you up, but they're missing essential nutrients like calcium, vitamin D, and protein that keep bones strong and muscles ready for action. Enter nutrient-rich foods: fresh fruits, veggies, whole grains, lean proteins. Think of them as the maintenance crew your body needs to stay resilient.

Here's a pro tip: instead of thinking about what you "shouldn't" eat, focus on sneaking in more of the good stuff. Add a handful of greens to your meal, trade one soda for a glass of water, or try a new veggie each week. Little swaps build up overtime to a diet that supports a strong, resilient body.

Skimping on Sleep: The Silent Sabotage

Ah, sleep. It's the ultimate reset button for our bodies, a natural miracle drug that costs absolutely nothing. Yet, who hasn't thought, "I'll just stay up a little longer..." only to feel like a zombie the next day? When we regularly sacrifice sleep, our bodies start to suffer. Muscles don't recover, our mental clarity takes a nosedive, and our immune system gets sluggish, opening us up to illness.

Think of sleep as your body's nightly maintenance team. When you skimp on it, you're cutting out vital time for repairs. Over time, this "sleep debt" adds up, weakening muscles, bones, and even our motivation to stay active. Not to mention, poor sleep can dampen mood and energy levels, making it even harder to stick to the habits that prevent frailty. So, commit to those seven to nine hours of sleep and make it non-negotiable. Just like you wouldn't skip a dentist's appointment, don't skip on your ZZZs.

Stress and Its "Subtle" Side Effects

If stress were a person, it'd be that overbearing friend who never leaves you alone and keeps whispering terrible advice. Chronic stress doesn't just impact our mood; it affects everything from our immune system to our mental and physical resilience. Stress hormones like cortisol, when chronically elevated, can lead to muscle breakdown, weakened bones, and even cognitive decline.

And here's the catch: when we're stressed, we're more likely to make poor choices that fuel frailty, like reaching for junk food, skipping workouts, or skimping on sleep. It's a vicious cycle. So, what's the antidote? Find your personal stressbusters. Whether it's meditation, talking with friends, exercise, or a creative outlet like painting or writing, having a go-to strategy can help you keep that resilience intact.

The "Tomorrow" Mindset: Procrastination's Quiet Creep

"I'll start that exercise program next week" or "I'll eat better after the holidays" are classic phrases that many of us use. But here's the kicker: tomorrow never comes. Each time we push off positive changes, we're letting frailty inch a little closer. Over time, "later" becomes a habit in itself, and before you know it, the resilience we once took for granted has dwindled.

Building resilience is about creating habits today that pay off tomorrow. Start small, even if it's five minutes of activity, one healthy meal swap, or an early night here and there. The best part? Small changes snowball. A daily five-minute walk can become ten, then twenty. A handful of blueberries instead of chips becomes a routine. When you put "future you" first, you're creating a path that leads away from frailty.

Mindless Snacking: The Tiny Temptation Trap

Who hasn't reached for a quick snack only to realize they've emptied the whole bag? Snacking itself isn't the enemy, it's the mindless, nutrient-poor snacking that gets us. Chips, candy, or other processed foods might be satisfying for a moment, but over time, they add up to a diet low in essential vitamins and minerals.

Instead, turn snacking into a chance to sneak in more nutrients. Fresh fruit, nuts, yogurt, or veggies with hummus make excellent snack options that feed your body instead of just filling it. When we shift our focus to snacks that strengthen our bones and muscles, we're actively choosing a stronger, healthier future.

Ignoring the Social Scene: When Solitude Takes a Toll

It might not seem like a big deal to skip a few social gatherings, but regular isolation chips away at our resilience. Studies consistently show that people with strong social connections are less likely to experience frailty and more likely to live longer, healthier lives (13). The human need for connection goes beyond just friendship—it supports mental health, keeps us active, and even strengthens immunity. Whether it's calling a friend, joining a club, or volunteering, social interaction keeps us engaged, mentally sharp, and emotionally fulfilled. The antidote to frailty is not just physical or mental strength, it's a vibrant social network that makes life richer and more resilient.

The Bottom Line: Frailty Prevention Is a Habit-Building Game

Ultimately, avoiding frailty is about recognizing these sneaky habits and making small changes today that build resilience tomorrow. It's about shifting our mindsets from "just one more" to "just one less," from "maybe tomorrow" to "let's do this today." Every choice we make, no matter how small, contributes to the grand tapestry of our future health.

So, take it one step, snack, and stretch at a time. Celebrate the wins, forgive the slip-ups, and remember that building resilience is a journey—a journey worth every small effort along the way. After all, a resilient you are the best gift you can give your future self!

Frailty In Simple Terms: Physical, Cognitive, And Emotional Aspects

Imagine frailty as a complex web, woven together by physical, cognitive, and emotional threads that pull tighter over time, making you feel like you've lost some spring in your step, sharpness in your mind, and even that zest for life. Sure, frailty often starts with the body—but that's just one of the players in this all-too-real comedy of aging. So, let's go on a tour of the three less-than-fabulous amigos: tired muscles, forgetful brain, and moody mind. It's not just about one system going off the rails; it's about the whole concert of life hitting a few too many flat notes.

Physical Frailty: Not Just About Weak Muscles

When we think of frailty, we often picture the physical part: you don't quite have the energy to climb five flights of stairs, or the agility to hop out of bed without feeling like you might topple over. And that's because, yes, physical frailty is about the body's resilience or, as it begins to dwindle, its reluctance to keep up. Your muscles are a big part of this equation—strong muscles mean more than just lifting weights; they keep you balanced, help absorb shocks and give you stamina for everything from picking up your grandkids to catching the last train home.

Physical frailty is like your body's quiet rebellion, a subtle but determined protest where muscle strength dwindles, balance gets wobbly, and endurance feels like a distant memory. Think of it as the "I'm tired, can't we just take a nap?" part of your body's story. But it's not just about muscular strength. Bone density sneaks into the mix too, as bones start to lose their superpowers and become more like fragile artifacts than iron-clad warriors. Every physical system—from your joints to your bones, even to your heart—is part of this club. And when they band together in slow decline, everyday tasks that once seemed effortless start feeling like monumental challenges.

The fix isn't just about throwing in more weight training or marathon sessions. It's about staying active in a sustainable way that reminds your body it still has a role to play. Little bits of strength training, balance work, or even a daily walk can signal your muscles and bones to stay strong and agile, keeping that physical resilience around a little longer. Just think of each stretch, squat, or step as a mini protest against frailty.

Cognitive Frailty: When Your Brain Needs a Tune-Up

Then there's cognitive frailty. It's like that slightly unreliable car in the garage—works fine one day, stalls the next. As we age, our brains don't exactly throw in the towel, but they can get a bit glitchy. Forgetting where you put your phone or fumbling with someone's name might seem like quirky slips, but cognitive frailty is deeper. Imagine your brain's Wi-Fi connection getting just a bit patchier: it's not down entirely, but there are certainly moments where it stutters and lags, making it hard to multitask, focus, or recall names at speed.

Reaction time slows down, so that split-second judgment call when a soccer ball comes flying your way. That becomes more like a slow-motion decision, complete with a few extra seconds to process. Cognitive frailty isn't just about memory, though—it also taps into attention, decision-making, and even the ability to handle stress or organize tasks. It's the reason your "mental flexibility" feels a little less flexible and a bit more rigid.

So, what's to be done? Surprisingly, a lot. Keeping your mind active, learning new things, or even practicing old hobbies (yes, like Sudoku or knitting) can work wonders. Your brain is a bit like a muscle, too—the more you stretch it, the stronger it can stay. And since physical and cognitive health are closely linked, are all that movement you're doing for your muscles? That's helping your brain too, increasing blood flow and keeping those neural pathways a little clearer.

Emotional Frailty: The Overlooked Player

Ah, emotional frailty, the sleeper hit in the frailty game. Emotional health is the unsung hero that often goes unnoticed until it isn't there. This part of frailty is trickier to pin down because it's subtle, yet impactful. It's that sense of being less connected to the people around you, or a creeping feeling of isolation that can turn even the sunniest day into a grey one. As physical and cognitive resilience starts to slip, emotional health can too. It's like a domino effect; if you're physically struggling and mentally slowing down, feeling connected or uplifted becomes tougher.

Emotional frailty has a way of sneaking up on people. It's that gradual inclination to skip social gatherings because you're tired or the nagging feeling that maybe you just don't have the energy to engage with the world like you once did. And loneliness isn't just a sad feeling; it's actually a physiological burden, too. Studies show that chronic loneliness can elevate stress hormones, mess with immune function, and even accelerate cognitive decline (14-16). It's as if our brains and bodies are hardwired to need connection as a survival tactic, and without it, we start to fray around the edges.

So, what can you do? Combatting emotional frailty is all about finding ways to stay engaged with others and creating connections that lift you up. Whether it's joining a book club, calling friends regularly, or volunteering somewhere you're passionate about, staying socially connected feeds the soul and, surprisingly, fortifies the body and mind, too. Think of each coffee date or family gathering as emotional weightlifting—keeping your heart strong and ready for whatever life throws your way.

Frailty's relationship with chronic conditions, disabilities, and socio-economic factors is often overlooked. These interactions are key to understanding the aging population and developing better health strategies.

Frailty Is the Full Package

So, there it is—frailty as the trio of physical, cognitive, and emotional challenges (17). Each element intertwines with the others, so a problem in one area often spills over to the next. Physical limitations can dampen your mood; cognitive slips can make you feel less confident and more isolated; and emotional strain can lead to less motivation for staying active and alert.

But and this is a big "but", there's plenty you can do about it. Just as frailty is an ensemble cast, prevention is, too. A well-rounded approach keeps all parts of your body, brain, and mood — functioning at their best. So yes, while frailty might be a multi-headed hydra of aging, every step you take toward resilience can keep each of these pesky heads at bay.

Frailty and Chronic Conditions

Chronic conditions such as diabetes mellitus (DM), heart disease, and arthritis can speed up the onset of frailty in older adults (18-20). These conditions damage the body over time, making it harder for the body to recover from illnesses or injuries. When someone has a chronic illness, their body's ability to heal and bounce back becomes weaker, and this can lead to long-lasting effects like fatigue, muscle weakness, and difficulty carrying out everyday tasks. As a result, individuals with chronic conditions often find themselves less able to cope with physical stress, which increases their risk of becoming frail. For example, DM can disrupt blood flow, impair nerve function, and weaken muscle factors that all contribute to frailty. When an older person has both frailty and a chronic condition, managing the disease becomes even more challenging. This can result in worse health outcomes, a higher likelihood of complications, and a lower quality of life overall.

Frailty and Disabilities

Frailty and disability, whether physical or cognitive, are deeply intertwined (21, 22). They act both as consequences and risk factors for each other. When someone struggles with mobility or has trouble performing everyday tasks—like bathing, dressing, or cooking, their independence starts to decline. This loss of activity not only reduces quality of life but also triggers muscle weakness and weight loss, which are key clues of frailty.

On the cognitive side, conditions like dementia produce a similar problem. Cognitive impairments make it difficult to manage one's health, keep up with medical routines, or even make simple decisions. This increased vulnerability to frailty can further compromise their ability to maintain a healthy lifestyle.

The relationship between frailty and disability generates a vicious cycle. Frailty limits a person's ability to stay active and engage in self-care, which worsens physical disabilities. For instance, someone with limited mobility may become frail because they can't move as much, leading to further physical decline. This, in turn, makes it even harder for them to stay active, perpetuating the cycle of frailty and disability. Breaking this cycle is crucial to improving the health and independence of older adults.

Frailty and Socio-Economic Factors

Socio-economic factors play a significant role in how frailty develops and its impact (23, 24). Older adults from lower socio-economic backgrounds often have limited access to healthcare, nutritious food, and safe living environments, all of which are essential for healthy aging. Poor nutrition, inadequate housing, and lack of access to healthcare can lead to increased risks of frailty.

Social isolation is another key factor. Older adults living alone or with limited social networks are more likely to experience frailty. Without support, they may have difficulty managing their health, accessing resources, or staying physically active. Financial constraints can also limit their ability to afford medications or treatments that could slow frailty progression.

Why This Matters

The combination of frailty, chronic conditions, disabilities, and socio-economic factors creates a complex web of challenges for older adults. It's not just one factor that contributes to poor health outcomes but how they all intersect. A person with frailty and a chronic illness like heart disease, who lives in an isolated, low-income area, may face a higher risk of hospitalizations, falls, and disability.

Understanding these interactions can help in designing targeted interventions. It's essential to consider not just the frailty of an individual but also how their environment, their health conditions, and their access to resources affect their overall well-being. Only then can we create effective strategies to improve health outcomes and quality of life for aging populations.

Frailty Over Time—The Slippery Slope

Frailty isn't something that shows up one day and knocks on your door like an unwelcome dinner guest. No, it's more like that neighbour who borrows your rake once and just keeps coming back until you've practically handed over your whole shed. Frailty starts subtly, sneaks around in the background, and if you're not careful, it settles in. Here's a glimpse of what frailty might look like over the decades if you decide to ignore all the good advice about keeping active, eating well, and managing stress. This is the "what-not-to-do" guide to aging gracefully (or, rather, ungracefully).

In Your 20s: Setting the Stage with Poor Choices

Your 20s are a time of invincibility, right? You're strong, healthy, and can stay up all night without repercussions. Well, that's what your youthful metabolism and relatively high energy levels lead you to believe. This is when frailty begins to stake its claim, even if it's not obvious yet. Sit all day on your couch with chips and binge-watch every show under the sun? Check. Rely on takeout for most meals? Double-check. Choose a weekend of partying over a weekend of rest? Absolutely. After all, you're young, and your body will bounce back… or so you think.

Here's the reality: the choices you make in your 20s lay down the foundation for your future self. Imagine your body is a house, and each pizza and late night is like leaving a tiny crack in the foundation. Sure, it's not causing issues now, but fast forward a decade or two, and those small cracks start adding up. When you sit all day and skimp on sleep, those essential body-building blocks— muscles, joints, even brain cells—start wearing down. So, if you're treating your body like a 24/7 snack bar and skipping workouts? Frailty is already sending you a "see you later" note, waiting to cash it in down the line.

In Your 30s: The Subtle Signs Start to Show

You've hit your 30s, and life is happening. Between work, social obligations, even a family, you're in the thick of it. Exercise? It's harder to squeeze in. Healthy eating? Who has time to cook? And sleep? Well, what's a few extra cups of coffee, right?

This is when the body, still resilient, starts sending subtle hints. It might be a little harder to bounce back after a late night, or you find yourself getting winded going up a few flights of stairs. You're not frail by any means, but there's a shift—your body is starting to whisper, "Hey, take it easy on me!" The extra slice of cake, the skipped workout, and the nights hunched over your laptop aren't doing any favors. Those muscle aches and tightness in the shoulders. That's your body's way of reminding you to stretch, move, and drink water.

The good news is, you still have plenty of time to shape things up and make some healthy habits a natural part of your day. Start listening to the whispers, though, because they'll only get louder if ignored.

In Your 40s: Frailty Gets a Little Louder

Welcome to your 40s, where if you've been letting things slide, your body is no longer whispering, it's clearing its throat. This is the decade where subtle inconveniences from your 30s start becoming annoyances. Your flexibility? Not what it used to be. Your stamina? Well, let's just say you might need an extra rest day after a Saturday hike. And your mind? Occasionally, you forget where you put the keys or blank on someone's name, and you chalk it up to being "just one of those days."

It's your brain and body both sending little reminders that they need TLC. Without the cushion of good habits, muscles lose strength faster than you'd like, and joints start creaking. Frailty isn't glaring at you yet, but it's keeping a closer eye. This is the decade when stretching becomes a necessity, where you start noticing what happens when you skip out on sleep for more than a night or two. If you let the stress of work and family take over without balancing it with healthy habits, you'll notice how quickly resilience starts to wear down.

In Your 50s: Frailty Starts Waving a Flag

Ah, the 50s—a time of wisdom, growth, and a few more aches and pains. If you've consistently neglected your body's needs, it's going to start showing up more noticeably here. Muscles are weaker, joints are a little stiffer, and suddenly, you're all too familiar with the word "creak." The stiffness that used to disappear after a few minutes in the morning now seems to linger, and stairs have become something to approach with more caution than confidence.

The brain starts showing some signs, too—an occasional word might slip your mind, and multi-tasking doesn't come as easily. The "senior moments" that were cute in your 40s are now a little more frequent. You might find yourself avoiding physical activity because it's just plain harder, and if you haven't built a strong foundation of resilience, even routine activities start to feel like challenges.

Now, if you've been diligent about healthy habits, things might not be so daunting, but frailty becomes a very real possibility if you haven't. This is a wake-up call, but not all hope is lost. The body and mind can still adapt and improve; it's just a little more work than it would've been a couple of decades back.

In Your 60s and Beyond: Frailty Comes Knocking

Your 60s, 70s, and beyond should be a time to reap the rewards of a well-lived life. Ideally, if you've taken care of your body, you're still moving comfortably, engaging in activities you love, and savouring time with family and friends. But if frailty has been silently building over the years, this is when it's going to make itself known.

By now, muscles are naturally weaker, bones a bit more brittle, and the balance you once took for granted might be a little shakier. Joints, deprived of flexibility and strength, start to protest with every step. If you've ignored good sleep, nutritious foods, and regular exercise, you might find everyday tasks more tiring and feel the urge to sit things out more often. The "brain fog" becomes a little thicker, and memory slip-ups are a bit more common, not to mention that resilience to illness takes a noticeable hit.

This might sound bleak, but it doesn't have to be! Even at this stage, movement, nourishing food, and a bit of mindfulness can make a difference. A lot of people, with a bit of effort, stay sharp and spry well into their 70s and beyond. But if you haven't heeded the earlier signs and let frailty creep in, the slope to staying active and healthy becomes quite steep.

The Moral of the Frailty Story

Frailty isn't something that appears overnight. It's more like a debt, collecting tiny amounts of interest from every poor habit or moment of neglect. The good news? Just like a savings account, small deposits over time can build up resilience, keeping frailty at bay. No matter what your age, you can always start making those small changes, building your resilience, and preparing for a future where you're still moving, still engaged, and very much not frail. So, swap that next "oh, I'll work out tomorrow" with a quick stretch or a walk—you'll thank yourself later!

Prevention Is Key—The Anti-Frailty Blueprint

Alright, so let's talk about prevention—because here's the secret: when it comes to aging gracefully, prevention is the real VIP. Think of it as giving your future self a giant hug and a high-five. You might be picturing frailty as some vague thing you'll deal with "someday," but the truth is, it's the small, intentional steps you take now that make the biggest difference in steering clear of frailty's grasp later on. And no, we're not talking about signing up for ultra-marathons or swearing off dessert forever (life's too short, right?). Prevention is about setting up a sustainable, enjoyable way of living that helps you feel strong, capable, and resilient—for decades to come.

Imagine frailty prevention as a "choose your own adventure" story where each little choice you make adds up. Want to keep hiking, dancing, or even gardening in your golden years? Those tiny habits you start now are like seeds you're planting, and the harvest is a future full of energy and zest. Think of your body and mind as a lifelong investment, and with the right strategies, they'll yield lifelong returns.

In this section, we're building an anti-frailty blueprint—no hammering or welding required! We're going to show you how little tweaks to your daily routine can have a big impact. This is the ultimate roadmap to avoid frailty—detouring you past "Creaky Joint Junction" and "Brain Fog Boulevard." Instead, we'll set you up for a scenic route through "Healthy Muscle Heights" and "Mental Clarity Meadows." Each chapter will give you practical, easy-to-implement advice on staying strong, energized, and ready for anything, from travel and hobbies to simply enjoying life.

Let's start with the movement: yes, exercise is key, but don't worry if you're not into hours at the gym or training for triathlons. Regular movement—whether that's a walk, a gentle jogging session, or dancing around the kitchen—is the ultimate anti-frailty tonic. We'll explain how a little bit of regular physical activity, customized to your taste, can boost bone health, keep your muscles active, and even help prevent falls. And if you're still skeptical, just remember this:

when it comes to movement, the best exercise is the one you enjoy enough to keep doing.

Next up is diet, and here's where we get to banish any fears of forever giving up your favorite treats. Healthy eating doesn't have to mean kale smoothies and "superfoods" 24/7. Instead, think of nutrition as building a foundation with foods that support your bones, muscles, and mind. There's even room for pizza and a little dessert! The key is balance: you'll learn how to prioritize nutrient-rich foods that keep your body humming along, so you're fuelling up with what you need while still indulging in what you love.

Then, there's the importance of social connections. Frailty prevention isn't just about physical health; it's about mental and emotional wellness, too. Loneliness and isolation can have real consequences for our health, so in this chapter, we'll dive into why it's essential to keep up with friends, make new connections, and even say "yes" to that social event you've been considering. Not only does staying socially engaged ward off frailty, but it also brings more fun into your life, something we can all benefit from.

We'll also talk about keeping your mind sharp. Frailty might try to sneak in through forgetfulness and mental fatigue, but with a few brain-boosting habits, you can keep it at bay. Activities that engage your mind—whether that's reading, learning a new language, or solving puzzles—build cognitive resilience. You don't have to turn into a genius overnight; just choose hobbies that challenge your brain and keep your neurons firing on all cylinders.

And, of course, let's not forget about managing stress. Chronic stress wears us down physically and mentally, making it easier for frailty to creep in. In this section, you'll learn why managing stress is like adding armor to your anti-frailty toolkit. We'll explore easy, fun ways to de-stress, from practicing mindfulness to taking up a creative hobby or just letting yourself enjoy a good laugh. Because sometimes, he best anti-frailty prescription is simply a little bit of joy.

So, think of this blueprint as your personal guide to a future that's full of energy, joy, and resilience. Yes, aging is inevitable, but by putting in a little effort now, you can age in a way that lets you keep doing the things you love, with the people you love. The best part? Each small step adds up to big rewards, creating a future where frailty isn't even on the radar. Whether you're 30, 50, or 70, it's never too early (or too late!) to start building a life that's vibrant, strong, and frailty-free.

Muscle Health—Body's Secret Weapon Against Frailty

Alright, let's dive deeper into why muscles are the unsung heroes of aging and how to keep them thriving—because believe it or not, our muscles are the key to aging well and dodging the dreaded F-word (frailty, which is).

First things first: muscles don't just sit there looking pretty (though yes, they can make you look rather fit in your favorite outfit). They are your very own, built-in support system that springs into action whenever you need them. Muscles are what allow you to run, jump, lift, carry, climb, and do all the other things that make life dynamic. Think of muscles as the fuel injectors of your body, powering up every movement, stabilizing every balance challenge, and keeping your bones safely padded and supported. Without muscle health, even the simplest things—like getting out of a chair or carrying groceries—can start to feel like scaling a mountain.

The Magic of Muscles Beyond the Mirror

But muscle health goes far beyond physical strength and appearance. Muscle tissue plays a powerful role in our inner workings, too. Muscles are actively involved in our metabolism, which means that when they're healthy and active, they help burn calories even at rest. This becomes especially important as we age because a healthy metabolism helps regulate our body weight and fend off chronic diseases like diabetes mellitus. Plus, muscle tissue is essential in regulating blood sugar— acting like a sponge to soak up glucose from the bloodstream, which keeps blood sugar levels in check. Think of muscles as the quiet but effective "thermostats" of your body, keeping you at the ideal temperature for good health.

And let's not forget the energy boost! When your muscles are in good shape, they're essentially mini power plants that give you the stamina you need to tackle daily activities without tiring them out by noon. Healthy muscles help maintain endurance, allowing you to stay active, keep up with family and friends, and avoid the dreaded "midday slump." So, while muscles may not get as much attention as, say, heart health, they are the hidden allies working behind the scenes to keep you thriving.

What's at Stake: The Silent Sneak of Sarcopenia

Let's get real for a moment. Starting around age 30, we begin to experience gradual muscle loss—an ominous process called "sarcopenia." This isn't just some vague term scientists toss around; it's the gradual thinning of our muscle tissue that, if left unchecked, chips away at our strength and mobility. The culprit? A mix of factors like reduced physical activity, hormonal changes, and not-so- great nutritional choices.

If this sounds daunting, it kind of is—especially if you let sarcopenia have free rein. But the good news? This whole muscle-losing situation isn't set in stone. With the right habits and mindset, you can hold on to a substantial amount of muscle strength well into your later years, keeping that vibrant, capable "you" alive and kicking.

Working Your Muscles: It's Easier (and More Fun) Than You Think

Think keeping your muscles healthy means signing up for an intense gym membership or spending hours lifting heavy iron? Not necessarily! There are so many ways to work out that they aren't about becoming the next bodybuilder; they're simply about keeping your muscles activated and engaged so they stay put.

Resistance training, for instance, is one of the best ways to combat muscle loss, and you don't need fancy equipment to do it. Resistance bands, water bottles, even your own body weight can do the trick. Exercises like squats, lunges, and push-ups can be done anywhere and provide amazing benefits. And, if lifting weights isn't your style, try activities that blend cardio with muscle- strengthening movements like yoga, Pilates, or even dance classes (hello, salsa dreams!).

Plus, every little bit counts. Gardening, walking your dog, playing with your kids or grandkids — these activities all engage your muscles and help maintain your strength. If you're moving and occasionally challenging those muscles with something a little tougher, they'll continue to serve you well.

The Power of Protein: Muscles' Best Friend

Here's the scoop on another muscle-building tip: protein. Protein is essential for muscle repair and growth, and as we age, our bodies actually need a bit more of it to maintain the muscle mass we have. Now, before you picture yourself chomping down on a steak after every workout, let's talk balance. Protein doesn't have to be all about meat. Lean meats, yes, but also plant-based sources like beans, lentils, tofu, and nuts offer high-quality protein. Even dairy can be a great source (cue a delicious Greek yogurt bowl or a satisfying cheese snack).

Incorporating protein into each meal can help keep muscles in good shape and aid in recovery after physical activity. Plus, it helps curb that hunger that often sneaks up when you're trying to cut down on unnecessary snacks. And no, that doesn't mean saying goodbye to your favorite treats—it just means balancing them with muscle-friendly protein.

Muscle Maintenance Is the New Fountain of Youth

Imagine your muscles as a lifelong investment. Each time you go for a brisk walk, take a yoga class, or lift that carton of milk just a little bit more purposefully, you're adding to this "muscle bank." In turn, your muscles pay you back by giving you the strength to stay independent, energetic, and physically capable as you age.

So, here's the takeaway: muscle health isn't just a "nice-to-have"—it's a cornerstone of healthy aging. Whether it's hauling heavy groceries, chasing after grandkids, or yes, maybe even salsa dancing under the stars, your muscles make it all possible. And the best part? You don't need to be an athlete or spend hours sweating it out. You just need to keep moving, add in a little strength training, and fuel up with muscle-loving foods. Because a resilient, capable body is built over time—one step, one stretch, one meal at a time.

Strength-Building Activities That Can Be Done At Any Age.

Alright, it's time to unleash the mighty muscles! No, this isn't a call to become a bodybuilder or bench-press your sofa (unless that's your thing). Strength is for everyone, and these activities will keep you feeling vibrant and strong no matter your age—and they don't even require a gym. With a little creativity and commitment, you can turn about any space into your personal fitness hub. So, lace up those sneakers, grab some water, and get ready to learn how to make strength-building a natural, feel-good part of your day-to-day life.

Bodyweight Exercises: The Original Fitness Hack

Bodyweight exercises are like that trusty old friend you can count on—they're simple, effective, and always around. No need for equipment or complex setups; your body is the equipment! Just think push-ups, squats, lunges, and planks. Don't let their simplicity fool you. These moves can give you serious muscle power.

Take 'squats', for example. With each rep, you're firing up your glutes, quads, hamstrings, and even your core. Try doing squats while you're waiting for the coffee to brew or during TV commercials. Before you know it, you'll have steel thighs, and your couch will become the most intimidating seat in the house. And then there's the classic 'push-up'. Sure, it's just pushing yourself off the ground, but each push-up works your arms, chest, and shoulders, creating a cascade of strength that radiates through your upper body.

If push-ups and squats sound too ambitious, no problem. Modify them! Wall push-ups and chair-assisted squats are gentle ways to start, giving you all the benefits without strain. Start small, work up gradually, and soon you'll be conquering more reps than you ever thought possible.

Resistance Bands: Your Pocket-Sized Gym

Meet the humble resistance band—a stretchy, portable miracle that transforms any room into a gym. These bands come in different levels of resistance, so whether you're a newbie or a pro, there's one for you. Slip one around your thighs for leg lifts or use it for 'arm curls' and 'shoulder presses'. Think of them as mini personal trainers, adding a bit of challenge to familiar moves.

What's wonderful about resistance bands is that they let you control the intensity. For a full workout, you could start with a quick 'glute bridge' session by placing the band above your knees, lying down, and lifting your hips. Feel the burn? Good. Now add a 'bicep curl' using a longer band anchored under your foot. This is strength-building without the gym sweat or intimidating machines—and yes, it counts!

Everyday Activities as Exercise: Sneaky Strength in Disguise

Who says you have to change into workout clothes to get a workout? Everyday chores can be strength-building champions in disguise. 'Carrying grocery bags?' That's arm day right there. 'Walking up a flight of stairs?' You're working out your legs and glutes. Think of it as "incidental exercise"—a fancy way of saying that even the mundane can make you stronger if you give it the chance.

Take a closer look at those repetitive household tasks. 'Gardening', for example, requires squatting, pulling, and lifting—all the moves of a full-body workout. Same goes for 'vacuuming' or 'cleaning windows.' By engaging your muscles and moving with purpose, you're doing far more than cleaning, you're also boosting your muscle strength, balance, and stamina. No gym required!

Yoga and Pilates: Calm Yet Powerful

Picture this: you're balancing on one foot in a tree pose, finding your center, while gently challenging every stabilizing muscle in your body. That's yoga—a workout that isn't just for flexibility but for full-body strength, too. Many yoga poses like 'warrior' or 'plank' build both endurance and stability, turning you into a powerhouse of quiet resilience. Plus, it's an ideal choice for any age, helping keep your joints limber and your core muscles engaged without needing fancy equipment or a monthly gym membership.

'Pilates', on the other hand, focuses on what enthusiasts lovingly call the "powerhouse"—the muscles of your core, including your abs, lower back, and hips. While it might seem slow, don't let it fool you; Pilates can be as intense as weightlifting when done right. And it's incredibly gentle on the joints, which makes it perfect for those who want a low-impact workout that delivers big results.

All you need is a mat and a little floor space. These exercises are your path to graceful, toned strength that sneaks up on you with each session, keeping you balanced, flexible, and strong without you even realizing it.

Dance Like No One's Watching

When was the last time you put on your favorite song and just 'danced'? Not only is dancing a great cardio workout, but it also builds strength. The effort it takes to hold yourself steady while moving to the beat works your core, legs, and arms in a fun, feel-good way.

Dancing also has the added benefit of improving coordination, which is key for keeping you spry as you age. Try a 'twist-and-turn routine' in your living room or join a Zumba class and groove along to upbeat tunes. This is an all-ages, feel-good way to sneak in strength training while having an absolute blast.

Balance Exercises: Because Balance is Strength Too

Balance is one of those underrated skills that doesn't get enough attention until we really need it. And guess what? Good balance is also a form of strength! Simple balance exercises like 'standing on one leg' or 'walking heel-to-toe' are fantastic ways to engage your core and stabilizing muscles.

Start with something as easy as 'tree pose' in yoga or try lifting one leg while brushing your teeth (just don't accidentally poke yourself with the toothbrush!). Improving balance today means staying more active, mobile, and resilient in the future, helping you avoid slips and falls.

Stair Climbing: The Stealth Strength Workout

Stairs: the unsung heroes of strength training. Walking up and down stairs isn't just good for cardio; it also gives your calves, glutes, quads, and hamstrings a real workout. You don't have to do a full stair sprint to reap the benefits, either. Just make it a habit to take the stairs wherever you go, and you'll be squeezing in a mini workout multiple times a day.

If you're looking for a challenge, try skipping a step for added glute and quad engagement. Not only will you build strength, but you'll also be doing your heart a favor. The beauty of stair climbing is that it's readily available and free, making it the perfect workout that just "steps" right into your day. Playtime Activities: Fun with Benefits

Remember how fun it was to play as a kid? Turns out, those playful activities are strength-building, too. Games like 'throwing a frisbee', 'catching a ball', or 'hiking' aren't just enjoyable; they're natural ways to engage muscles without even feeling like you're working out.

Playing with kids or pets can also sneak strength training into your day. Try lifting a toddler for a full-body boost (those little ones are heavier than they look!) or play tug-of-war with your dog for an arm workout. The point here is to have fun while keeping your body strong.

Small But Mighty: The Power of Consistency

Now that we've covered so many options, here's the real secret to strength-building: consistency. It's the little, consistent habits that stack up to make a big difference. Find what you enjoy, whether it's bodyweight exercises, gardening, or a weekly dance session, and make it part of your routine. Because when it comes to building strength, showing up regularly matters way more than going all-out on occasion.

So, here's to a future filled with strength, resilience, and energy. Embrace these exercises, and watch how your body responds with more balance, flexibility, and endurance. Whether you're lifting grocery bags, striking a yoga pose, or just standing tall, remember—you're building the kind of strength that'll carry you through life's adventures with vigor and vitality. And that's worth every squat, stretch, and dance move.

"Use It Or Lose It": Muscles, Joints, And Bones

Alright, picture this: your muscles, joints, and bones are back at the roundtable meeting inside your body, but this time, they're holding an intervention. The muscles, naturally the boldest of the group, begin, "Look, we're all about keeping things moving, but we've been sitting dormant for way too long. We're supposed to lift and carry, not rust!" The joints nod in agreement, chiming in, "We're supposed to help you reach, stretch, and explore the world—not just pivot from the fridge to the couch!" Meanwhile, the bones, a bit stiff themselves, declare with a touch of exasperation, "We're the structure here—the literal framework! But without regular activity, we're becoming as brittle as an old newspaper!"

It's time to face facts: if you don't give your muscles, joints, and bones the attention they deserve, they'll drift apart like a neglected friend group that hasn't caught up in years. It's a classic case of "use it or lose it," and they're all here to remind you of their specific, highly relatable needs. Imagine it as a group chat that's gone silent for too long; if nobody keeps it active, it fades into oblivion, just like your muscles when you start skipping the gym or your bones when they're starved for a good workout.

Muscles: The Powerhouses in Hibernation

First, let's chat about muscles, the powerhouses that tend to start pouting when ignored. Muscles thrive on attention, and if you're not giving them the stimulation they crave, they'll weaken faster than a Wi-Fi signal on a stormy day. Muscles are there for strength, for movement, for standing tall in the world! But leave them unattended, and they start dwindling, becoming less responsive, and sadly… a bit mushy. Yes, even muscles can lose their mojo if you don't use them regularly. And we're not just talking about biceps here; we mean the whole set, from the legs that carry you to the core that holds you upright.

Strength training is the ultimate pep talk for muscles. Each squat, lunge, and lift send a direct message: "Stay strong; we need you!" You don't need to be bench-pressing ridiculous weights or setting new gym records. Even light strength exercises, like lifting hand weights or using resistance bands, remind your muscles they're essential and loved. By keeping them engaged, you're ensuring they'll be there when you need to haul groceries, dance at weddings, or simply get out of a chair with grace.

Bones: The Backbone of It All, Literally

Bones, our often-overlooked heroes, are next. Imagine them like the reliable but underappreciated friend who's always there, keeping everything steady and together, even when you forget to send a thank-you text. Bones are the framework, the scaffolding upon which the rest of you is built. And while they might seem tough, they're not invincible, especially without a regular dose of weight-bearing activity.

When you lift weights, whether it's a dumbbell or a grocery bag, it's not just your muscles getting the workout. Bones respond to this pressure by reinforcing themselves, making sure they're strong enough to handle any load you throw away. This process, called "bone remodelling," keeps them dense and resilient. Think of it like giving your bones a little reminder: "Hey, we've got some work to do here!" Weight-bearing exercises like squats, lunges, or even just brisk walking are ways to keep your bones in top shape. You're telling them, "Stay strong, stay solid!" so they're prepared to handle life's bumps and tumbles without becoming fragile.

Skipping out on these exercises, on the other hand, is like leaving them unread messages; they get the hint that they're not needed, and they start to slack off. And over time, this leads to that dreaded brittleness—a dangerous outcome, as it increases the risk of fractures and falls.

Joints: Flexibility Is the Secret to Longevity

Let's not forget the joints, the flexible friends that make sure you can reach, bend, twist, and stretch to your heart's content. Unlike bones, joints don't get tougher with impact; they get happier with movement. But the kind of movement they like is smooth, gentle, and stretchy—like a morning yoga class, not an intense sprint up a mountain. Joints love low-impact activities that keep them lubricated and limber, whether that's yoga, tai chi, or a daily stretching routine.

When you skip out on these, joints become about as cooperative as a rusty hinge. They stiffen, lose their range of motion, and may start popping or creaking, giving you that unmistakable "I'm getting old" sound effect every time you stand up. Daily stretching and flexibility exercises can work wonders, though. Even small moves, like rolling your wrists or doing gentle neck stretches, keep them happy. And don't skip out on balance exercises! Balancing one foot, or trying simple stability moves, activates the muscles around your joints, adding a layer of protection against unexpected trips and falls.

The Trio in Action: Why They're Better Together

When muscles, bones, and joints are all strong and happy, it's like a harmonious orchestra that just makes life easier. You move with ease, you're resilient against falls, and even everyday tasks seem lighter. But ignore one member of the trio, and things get out of sync. Weak muscles can't support strong bones, stiff joints can't follow a flexible body's lead, and brittle bones don't stand a chance if muscles aren't there to cushion a fall.

Think of it this way: every skipped workout, every hit of the snooze button instead of taking that morning walk, every extra hour on the couch is a silent memo to your body that says, "Hey, let's just take it easy." But over time, taking it easy translates into losing muscle tone, bone density, and joint flexibility—leading to frailty and that creaky feeling you might remember from older relatives. Commit to regular activity, and you're reminding your muscles, bones, and joints to stay ready and resilient.

Movement as a Daily Ritual

Embracing the motto "use it or lose it" doesn't mean you need to become a gym regular or start intense training. Sometimes, it's about incorporating small, daily moments of movement. Walking around the block, taking the stairs, reaching for something on a high shelf, or even doing a little dance while cooking are simple reminders to your body that you're still in action mode. It's the little moments that add up, gradually reinforcing the trio's resilience and keeping you agile and strong.

When you're getting your daily dose of movement, think of it as maintenance—like watering a plant or tuning up a car. It's how you keep the whole system running smoothly, because if you don't use it, you'll lose it, whether you're 30 or 80. It might sound a little harsh, but it's an invitation to stay connected to your body, to celebrate its ability to move, stretch, and adapt. So go on, take a stretch break, lift a weight, or go for a walk, and keep that trio working as the dream team they're meant to be.

Bone Health And Its Role In Physical Resilience

Absolutely, let's dig deeper into the marvels of bone health—think of this as a TED Talk your bones would give if they could talk!

Let's face it: our bones are seriously underrated. While the heart gets all the love for pumping blood and the brain gets kudos for, well, making us conscious humans, bones work quietly behind the scenes, keeping us from becoming a heap on the floor. Imagine, for a second, that you're a jellyfish— beautiful in the ocean, but a nightmare on land. Thankfully, bones spare us from this floppy fate by giving us structure, allowing us to dance, climb, and survive our clumsy attempts at DIY projects.

The Marvels of Bone Structure and Function

Bones are like scaffolding for your entire body, but they're way cooler than any metal framework. A baby starts life with about 270 bones, but as they grow, some bones fuse, leaving the average adult with 206 sturdy pieces. And no, this doesn't make them like building blocks that stick together permanently, bones are dynamic, constantly regenerating to keep up with life's demands. There's something oddly poetic about bones breaking down and rebuilding throughout our lives, as if they're taking part in their own daily spa treatment, getting rid of old, worn-out cells and making way for fresh, new ones.

Each bone is uniquely designed for its role. Your femur, for example, isn't just there to look good on an X-ray. It's thick, dense, and perfectly crafted to bear the weight of the body. Meanwhile, the sophisticated vertebrae in your spine forms a flexible column that can twist, bend, and bear loads— all while housing and protecting your spinal cord, the body's superhighway for nerve signals. Even the tiniest bones, like the three little ones in your ear (the hammer, anvil, and stirrup), play a part in our survival, translating sound waves so we can pick up everything from the gentle hum of conversation to the telltale hiss of a snake in the grass.

Bone Remodelling: The Lifelong Construction Zone

Now, here's where things get interesting. Bones aren't static. They're a construction site that never closes, constantly undergoing a process called remodelling. It's like having an invisible team of builders and renovators—osteoclasts and osteoblasts—who work tirelessly to ensure your bones are strong and functional. Osteoclasts handle demolition, breaking down old or damaged bone. Then osteoblasts come in to rebuild with fresh materials, ensuring that your skeletal frame stays as strong as ever. This cellular give-and-take keeps bones adaptable, ready to fortify where stress is highest and repair where fractures threaten.

In fact, when you exercise, your bones "listen" to the pressure, and, in response, the osteoblasts get to work, reinforcing and thickening the bone tissue in areas that need more strength. It's like a personalized strength-training program for your skeleton, no gym membership required.

This is why astronauts, who float around in zero-gravity environments, have to work extra hard to keep their bones from becoming soft as butter. Without the resistance of gravity, their bones lose density. For the rest of us, all it takes is regular movement and some occasional weight-bearing exercise to give our bones the boost they need.

Calcium and Bone Health: The Dynamic Duo

Now, we can't talk about bone health without mentioning calcium—the Beyoncé to bones' Destiny's Child. Calcium is the mineral that hardens bones, making them strong enough to withstand everything from marathon runs to epic couch potato marathons. Your bones serve as a storage bank for calcium, ready to release it when other parts of your body need it. If your blood's calcium level drops too low, your bones will "donate" some of their stores to keep things in balance. Talk about being a team player!

But bones need more than just calcium to stay strong. They also rely on other nutrients like vitamin D, which helps your body absorb calcium. Think of vitamin D as calcium's VIP pass—it's what gets the mineral into your bloodstream in the first place. That's why soaking up a little sunlight or eating foods fortified with vitamin D is essential. And remember, bones are not picky eaters: they also crave magnesium, vitamin K, and even a little protein to stay in tip-top shape.

Bones: The Ultimate Shock Absorbers

Not only are bones strong, but they're also excellent shock absorbers. Each time you leap, run, or even just walk, your bones handle all the impact with grace. Picture it: every time you land a jump, whether it's on a trampoline or just hopping off a curb, your bones and joints spring into action, distributing and absorbing the force. This shock absorption isn't just about comfort, it's about resilience. Your bones work in tandem with cartilage (the body's cushioning material) to prevent wear and tear on other tissues, helping you stay agile and active.

When bones weaken, however, things go south quickly. A bone with reduced density is more prone to fractures and breaks, especially during high-impact activities or, let's face it, the occasional fall while trying to grab something from the top shelf. A fragile skeleton limits movement and independence, which is why keeping bones strong is essential for long-term physical resilience.

Bones and Balance: Staying Upright, One Step at a Time

Speaking of independence, bones are central to balance, too. Strong bones support good posture and stable movement. When your bones are in top shape, your muscles, ligaments, and tendons work in harmony to keep you upright and coordinated. But as bones lose density, posture suffers, and it can become more challenging to stay balanced. Weak bones lead to compensatory changes in how we walk and stand, which, over time, increase the risk of falls.

Picture this: a person with healthy bones and muscles walks with a confident stride, ready to tackle anything. Meanwhile, someone with fragile bones might move more cautiously, constantly on the lookout for obstacles, stairs, or stray marbles. This isn't just about appearances; it's about freedom and the ability to move without fear. Strong bones keep your sturdy, giving you the freedom to wander, explore, and, yes, even dance like no one's watching.

The Great Protector: Bones as Bodyguards

Aside from providing structure, bones are the bodyguards of our vital organs. The skull is like a fortress around the brain, absorbing impacts that might otherwise result in serious injury. The rib cage, meanwhile, acts as a protective cage for the heart and lungs, shielding these essential organs from all manner of knocks and bumps. Without these sturdy barriers, a simple fall or collision could lead to catastrophic damage.

Even your vertebrae work overtime as bodyguards, protecting the spinal cord. This delicate structure of nerves sends signals to and from the brain, allowing you to feel, move, and react. Without the shielding presence of the vertebrae, this crucial pathway would be extremely vulnerable. So next time you shrug, bow, or take a deep breath, thank your bones for the silent protection they offer every second of every day.

Keep Those Bones Busy: Exercise, Diet, and TLC

So, how do we keep this wonderful skeletal system healthy and resilient? It's all about balance: a mix of exercise, nutrition, and a little TLC. Weight-bearing exercises like walking, jogging, and even dancing stimulate bone growth, keeping bones dense and strong. And don't skimp on the stretching— flexibility is essential for a healthy, balanced skeleton.

Diet, of course, is also critical. While calcium and vitamin D are the stars, remember to feed your bones a variety of nutrients. Leafy greens, dairy products, nuts, and seeds are all bone-friendly choices. And if you really want to show your bones some love, make sure to stay hydrated. Water helps lubricate joints, reducing friction and wear overtime. Think of it as an all-natural bone moisturizer.

In brief: Bones Are the Quiet Heroes

In the end, bones are the unsung heroes of our bodies, working tirelessly to keep us upright, balanced, and resilient. They are more than just sturdy sticks holding us together; they're dynamic, protective, and essential for our well-being. By keeping our bones healthy, we're investing in a resilient future—one where we can keep moving, exploring, and thriving.

So next time you jump, lift, or even wiggle your toes, give a little nod of appreciation to your bones. After all, they're the original multitaskers, quietly holding everything together with strength, resilience, and style.

A Crash Course On Bone Density And How It Changes With Age

Alright, buckle up, because we're diving deep into the world of bone density, where your skeleton isn't just a bony structure but a complex, high-maintenance entity! Bone density isn't simply about "strong" versus "fragile"; it's all about how tightly packed the bone minerals are within the bone matrix. Think of it like a Jenga tower: when the blocks (or minerals) are neatly packed and stacked, it's sturdy. But if pieces start to go missing, well, let's just say your bones start looking like that tower right before it topples.

Your Golden Age of Bones: The Glorious Peak

Your bones, believe it or not, peak during your late teens to early twenties—a time when you're probably more concerned with surviving final exams than appreciating your superb skeletal structure. During this golden period, your bones are in their prime. Thanks to growth spurts, calcium, and a bit of genetic luck, your bone density levels reach their peak, as if your body decided to throw your skeleton the ultimate coming-of-age party. This is your body saying, "Enjoy these bones, kid. They'll never be quite this good again."

The Slow Decline: How Bone Density Changes Over the Years

For a couple of decades after your peak, bone density tends to hold steady, assuming you're living a reasonably healthy life. But by the time you hit your thirties, bone resorption—the fancy term for breakdown—starts to creep in, slowly surpassing the rate of bone formation. It's like your bones are finally admitting they can't keep up with the wear and tear forever. Imagine you're losing tiny grains of sand from your bones each day, making them just a bit less sturdy over time. This process is as unavoidable as getting gray hairs or realizing your knees make a suspicious cracking sound when you stand up too fast.

In your forties, the pace picks up a little more, as if your skeleton is easing into its "midlife crisis." Around this time, your body's internal bone-building contractors are off their game, while the demolition crew is working overtime. Without consistent effort in diet, exercise, and lifestyle, the bone density decline gains steam. This is when that Jenga tower we talked about earlier might start to feel a little wobbly, making you more susceptible to fractures and, eventually, osteoporosis if left unchecked.

The Menopause Effect: The Bone Density Plunge for Women

For women, the bone density game changes significantly post-menopause, and it all comes down to one word: estrogen. This hormone doesn't just regulate your menstrual cycle; it's also one of the best friends your bones will ever have. Estrogen helps keep bones dense, giving them structure and resilience. But after menopause, estrogen levels take a nosedive, and the bone density follows right behind. It's as if your bones got the memo, "No more baby-making duty," and decided to pack up shop. Women can lose up to 20% of their bone mass within the first five to seven years after menopause. The result? The skeleton doesn't quite have the spring in its step it once did, making it more prone to fractures and breaks.

Men don't think you're off the hook. While men maintain bone density longer than women, age-related bone loss catches up with you too. The process may be slower, but by the time men reach their seventies, the bone density decline starts to take a more significant toll.

How Can You Measure Your Bone Density?

So, how do you know if your bones are keeping it together? Meet the bone density test, or DEXA scan, your skeleton's version of a performance review. This non-invasive scan uses low-level X-rays to measure how tightly those minerals are packed in your bones, especially in your hips, spine, and wrists—areas that tend to go first if bone density takes a hit.

Here's how to read your T-score:

T-score of -1.0 or above: You're in the green! This is normal bone density, meaning you're still standing strong.

T-score between -1.0 and -2.5: Welcome to the "osteopenia" zone. Your bones are a bit less dense than they could be but haven't yet reached the fracture-prone stage.

T-score of -2.5 or lower: This is osteoporosis territory. Your bones are at higher risk for fractures, so it's time to act.

Knowing your T-score is crucial, like having a weather forecast for your bones. If you're hovering near the osteopenia or osteoporosis range, you can start making proactive changes before more serious complications arise. Think of it as your skeleton's way of dropping hints about what it needs from you.

Giving Your Bones Some Love: Tips for Long-Term Bone Health

Just like a prized houseplant that you've managed to keep alive, your bones need consistent TLC. Luckily, you don't need to overhaul your entire life to support your bone density. Here's the game plan:

Calcium and Vitamin D: They're the bread and butter of bone health. Aim for foods rich in calcium (dairy products, leafy greens, almonds) and get a little sun for vitamin D, or consider a supplement if you live in a cloudy climate. Vitamin D helps your body absorb calcium, making it a perfect sidekick in the quest for strong bones.

Weight-Bearing Exercise: Walking, dancing, jogging—any activity where your bones support your weight helps keep them strong. Strength training is especially effective; those weights do more than make your muscles pop. They create tiny "stressors" that encourage your bones to build density.

Quit Smoking and Limit Alcohol: Both can weaken bones, draining the calcium out of them like a sneaky sponge. Moderation is key if you want to keep your bones in tip-top shape.

Watch Out for Medications: Certain medications, like corticosteroids, can reduce bone density if taken long-term. Check with your doctor if you're on these to ensure you're doing everything possible to mitigate bone loss.

In the end, bone density isn't something that you can see or feel—until you break something, that is. That's why taking care of your bones now is such a worthwhile investment in your future self. Think of it as banking up strength and resilience for the years ahead so that you can continue to do the things you love, whether that's running marathons or simply running after grandkids.

So, embrace that DEXA scan, double-check your T-score, and treat your bones like the priceless support system they are. With a little attention and a few smart habits, you can keep that Jenga tower of bones standing strong, one brick at a time.

Nutrients, Activities, And Lifestyle Changes That Support Bone Health

Absolutely, let's dive into the bones of it all! Building up a strong skeleton isn't just for superheroes or gym fanatics. It's for anyone who wants to move, groove, and stay fracture-free well into their golden years. Think of it as investing in your own "skeletal 401 (k)." So, let's unpack the essential nutrients, rock-solid activities, and lifestyle changes that will help you sport a frame that could rival Iron Man.

Nutrients: The Building Blocks of a Bulletproof Skeleton

Calcium: The Cornerstone of Bone Strength

We all know calcium as the "it" mineral for bones, but it's more than just a buzzword your doctor throws around. Calcium is the main component of bone tissue, the actual stuff that forms the structure of your bones. Picture calcium as the bricks in a very tall, very important wall (your skeleton), making it a necessity, not a suggestion. Adults should aim for about 1,000 mg daily, or 1,200 mg if you're over 50, and it's available in dairy (yes, that means your morning latte counts), leafy greens, and fortified foods like orange juice and almond milk. The best part? Many of these foods are delicious, so it's really a win-win.

Vitamin D: The Sunshine Glue

Imagine if all those calcium bricks were piled up without any cement—one strong breeze (or slip) and down they go. Vitamin D is the body's mortar, helping absorb all that precious calcium and keeping it in place. Aim for about 600-800 IU per day, which you can get from a brisk stroll in the sunshine, fortified foods, or vitamin D-rich delights like salmon and eggs. Think of every sunbeam as a bone-boosting hug for your skeleton, making each minute outside feel productive (finally, guilt-free sunbathing!).

Protein: The Secret Ingredient for Bone Renewal

Bones aren't just hard slabs; they're dynamic, living tissues that need regular upkeep. Protein plays a crucial role here, as it provides the amino acids necessary for bone repair and maintenance. If calcium is bricks and vitamin D is the mortar, protein is the renovation crew, always repairing and remodelling. Get your fix from lean meats, legumes, beans, and nuts, which will work wonders in making your bones as strong as they can be. Plus, protein will give you a boost for all those bone- loving workouts we'll get into shortly.

Magnesium and Phosphorus: The Unsung Heroes

These two minerals don't get nearly the recognition they deserve. Magnesium helps regulate calcium levels and supports bone density, while phosphorus—naturally found in your bones—works with calcium to keep bones in top shape. Find these crucial nutrients in whole grains, nuts, seeds, and fish. Think of magnesium and phosphorus as the skeleton's security guards, quietly keeping everything balanced and functioning.

Activities: The Workout Plan Your Bones Have Been Waiting For

Weight-Bearing Exercises: Bones Love the Pressure

Weight-bearing exercises are any activities that make your body work against gravity, which helps stimulate new bone formation. This can mean anything from brisk walking and hiking to dancing and jogging. Imagine each step you take as a mini "strengthening session" for your bones, giving them the push they need to stay strong. Walking doesn't need to be Olympic-level either—every stroll around the neighborhood adds up. For bonus points, make it a habit and enjoy the scenery while you're at it.

Strength Training: The Bone Bulker

For bones, lifting weights is akin to adding reinforcements to an already sturdy structure. When you lift, you apply stress to your bones, prompting them to respond by adding more cells, which increases density. And you don't need gym membership or a bench press to see benefits —resistance bands, body-weight exercises, or even a couple of soup cans can do the trick. Every squat, lunge, or curl is a little investment in a fracture-proof future. Plus, strong muscles and strong bones go hand-in- hand, making it less likely you'll take a tumble in the first place.

Balance and Flexibility Exercises: Preventing the Downfall

It's hard to talk about bone health without addressing fall prevention. The best bones in the world won't help much if balance isn't part of the equation. Practices like yoga, tai chi, and specific balance drills not only make you more stable but also increase your agility. Think of these activities as giving your bones a "staying up" advantage. Imagine yourself as a serene yogi or graceful tai chi master—not only will you be calm and balanced, but your bones will also stay intact even on slippery floors.

Lifestyle Changes: Because Bones Need Love Too

Quit Smoking: Skeletons Don't Like Cigarettes

Smoking is like kryptonite for bones—it interferes with the body's ability to absorb calcium, weakens the structure, and even reduces bone mass. So, every puff makes bones just a little more brittle, setting you up for fractures down the road. It's a tough habit to kick, but your bones will thank you (as will your lungs, heart, and basically every other part of your body). If your goal is "Bones of Steel," it's best to give cigarettes the boot.

Limit Alcohol: Cheers to Moderation!

While that glass of wine might be enjoyable, heavy drinking can be harsh on your bones. Excessive alcohol consumption leads to bone loss and impedes calcium absorption, making them brittle. Moderate drinking (one drink a day for women, two for men) is the sweet spot for bone- friendly habits. So, savour your drink, but don't overdo it. Your bones will appreciate the moderation.

Maintain Healthy Weight: The Goldilocks Principle

A "just right" weight is ideal for bone health. Being underweight can mean bones aren't getting enough nutrients and are more likely to fracture, while being overweight adds unnecessary stress on bones and joints. A balanced diet paired with regular activity will keep your weight in the Goldilocks zone: not too heavy, not too light, but just right. It's all about finding that middle ground so your bones can support you through all of life's twists and turns.

Create a Fall-Proof Environment: Home Safety 101

Our bones love safety and creating a fall-proof environment at home can be your secret weapon. Remove tripping hazards like loose rugs, cords, or clutter; add non-slip mats to bathrooms and kitchens; and ensure every room is well-lit to avoid missteps. Grab bars in the shower and handrails on stairs are also a good idea. Think of it as building your very own "Bone-Safe Fortress." Your future self—and your skeleton—will be grateful for every precaution.

A Final Note: Build the Bones You Want to Grow Old With

All of this might sound like a lot, but building and maintaining strong bones is as simple as small, everyday habits adding up overtime. Calcium and vitamin D, a bit of sun, some weights, balance practice, and a bone-friendly home make a perfect recipe for longevity. And each healthy habit not only gives you a resilient skeleton but also boosts your energy, vitality, and even mood.

So, start today. Treat your bones like a prized possession, because they truly are—supporting you through every step, dance, hike, and adventure in life.

Cognitive Health And Physical Well-Being

Picture your brain as the conductor of a finely-tuned orchestra and your body as the musicians executing every note. When the conductor (your brain) is in sync with the musicians (your body), the harmony is breathtaking. But if one is offbeat or out of tune, the entire performance falters. Cognitive health and physical well-being are so intertwined that one's health directly impacts the other, resulting in either a beautiful, synchronized performance—or a chaotic one.

First off, let's talk about your brain's role in daily physical tasks. Contrary to what we might wish, your brain can't take a vacation and still expects your body to function optimally. It relies on the "machine" of your body to supply the essentials: oxygen, nutrients, and hydration. Picture these as the high-octane fuel keeping the conductor energized and alert. When you nourish your body well and stay active, it's like giving your brain a premium tune-up. Exercise and nutrition aren't just for bulking up muscles or looking fit; they are direct lines to optimizing cognitive performance. Think of it like upgrading your brain's processing power from an old-school modem to fiber-optic speeds.

Exercise: The Brain's Fountain of Youth

Now, here's the incredible thing about exercise: it doesn't just keep your muscles and joints in check; it actively nurtures your brain. Regular physical activity floods your brain with blood, delivering oxygen and nutrients to keep neurons firing efficiently. Research shows that exercise releases a substance called brain-derived neurotrophic factor (BDNF), which promotes the growth of new neurons, a process called neurogenesis. Imagine BDNF as a landscaper pruning and nourishing your brain's garden, ensuring every neural pathway is clear and vibrant.

Even better, exercise releases endorphins—those feel-good chemicals that make you feel invincible after a workout. Ever notice how a jog or a quick walk can leave you in a better mood? That's not just a psychological boost; it's your brain rewarding you for giving it a fresh supply of nutrients and oxygen. Over time, these neurochemical rewards help to reduce the risk of cognitive decline, acting like a shield against issues such as dementia.

Fuelling the Conductor: Nutrition's Role in Brain Health

Of course, even the best performance won't last if you're running on empty—or worse, on junk fuel. A balanced diet rich in fruits, vegetables, lean proteins, and healthy fats gives your brain the raw materials it needs to perform at its peak. Omega-3 fatty acids, for instance, are celebrated for their brain-boosting properties. Found in foods like salmon, walnuts, and flaxseeds, they support neuronal structure and protect against inflammation. Picture Omega-3s as the repair crew keeping the highways of your brain smooth and free of potholes.

Antioxidants from colorful fruits and veggies like berries, spinach, and carrots work like shields for your brain cells, protecting them from oxidative stress and free radical damage. Imagine them as bodyguards standing between your neurons and the harmful agents that can age and damage your brain. And let's not overlook hydration! Drinking enough water is essential, as even mild dehydration can impair concentration, short-term memory, and alertness. Just as an orchestra relies on precise timing and coordination, your brain relies on hydration to keep communication flowing smoothly.

The Brain-Body Connection: Why Sleep is Crucial

You might be tempted to skimp on sleep in today's fast-paced world, but sleep is vital for both body and mind. During those seven to nine hours of nightly rest, your brain is hard at work — consolidating memories, processing emotions, and, most importantly, detoxifying. Think of sleep as your brain's "night shift," where waste products are cleared out of neural passageways, readying your brain for another day. This process reduces the build-up of harmful proteins associated with Alzheimer's disease, so by catching those z's, you're keeping your brain's janitorial crew on task.

If you've ever been sleep-deprived, you know the consequences: foggy thinking, impulsivity, and slower reaction times. Studies have shown that chronic sleep deprivation can accelerate cognitive decline and exacerbate mental health issues like depression and anxiety (25, 26). So, next time you're tempted to stay up late binging on a new show, remember that a well-rested brain is a high-performing brain.

Mood Matters: Mental Health's Influence on Physical Health

Now, here's a fascinating twist: cognitive health doesn't just affect the brain but directly influences your body's stress response and immune function. When your brain is under constant stress, it signals the release of cortisol, the stress hormone. While cortisol can be helpful in short bursts, prolonged exposure weakens your immune system, disrupts sleep, and even slows digestion. Imagine having a nagging conductor who's constantly stressing the orchestra—after a while, the musicians would be exhausted and out of sync.

Cognitive health is vital for managing emotions and making healthy choices. A brain that's centered and resilient is better equipped to handle life's curveballs without spinning into a stress cycle. This is why practices that calm the mind, like mindfulness and meditation, are beneficial. They don't just help you find inner peace; they physically reduce stress hormones, balance your mood, and set the stage for a body that functions in harmony with a peaceful, alert mind.

The Dynamic Duo: Physical and Cognitive Health Working Together

Your brain and body are a dynamic duo, each one influencing and enhancing the other's performance. By taking care of your physical health—through exercise, nutrition, and sleep—you're giving your brain the resources it needs to function optimally. And by nurturing your mental and cognitive health, you're more likely to stick with the habits that keep your body strong, like avoiding that third slice of pizza and opting for a quick workout instead.

Next time you're lacing up your sneakers for a jog or picking up some leafy greens at the store, remember that you're not just boosting your physical fitness; you're feeding your brain, fortifying its resilience, and creating a solid foundation for a long, healthy life. In this symphony of life, cognitive and physical health are the instruments that, when well-tuned, play the harmonious melody of well-being. So, keep your conductor happy, fuel those musicians, and let the concert of your life play in full swing!

Simple Mental Exercises And Mindfulness Practices To Enhance Resilience

Alright, let's roll up our mental sleeves and dive deeper into the wonderful world of brain-boosting and resilience-building exercises. Who knew growing your resilience could be as fun as it is effective? Think of these practices as a mental spa day that offers your mind a bit of TLC, helps you keep calm, and keeps you laughing in the face of life's challenges.

Puzzle It Out (Because Your Neurons Need a Workout, too!)

Ever think of a crossword or a Sudoku puzzle as brain food? You should! These classic mental teasers not only sharpen your problem-solving skills, but they also keep your mind agile. And the best part? They're portable! Whip one out on the bus or while waiting for your coffee, and you're giving your brain a mini-gym session right there. If crossword clues start reminding you of cryptic advice from wise relatives, you're on the right track. And here's the bonus: solving puzzles boosts dopamine (the "feel-good" neurotransmitter), making you feel both accomplished and oddly blissed-out.

Learn Something New

Learning a new skill isn't just about impressing friends with an impromptu ukulele solo (though, let's face it, that's cool). Engaging in new activities builds fresh neural pathways, keeping your brain flexible and adaptable. Try your hand at painting, take up a dance class, or —why not—learn to juggle! Each new skill rewires your brain for resilience and mental agility. Not to mention, you'll get the bonus joy of saying, "I actually know a bit of Swahili!" at dinner parties.

Memory Games (or Never Lose Your Keys Again!)

Who knew that a little memory game could turn you into the household legend who never forgets where things are? Memory games, like the classic "matching pairs" or "Simon Says" are more than just nostalgia-inducing throwbacks to childhood—they strengthen your working memory and boost concentration. Plus, they're the ultimate friendly competition if you ever want to challenge friends or family. Even just setting small memory challenges for yourself, like recalling a grocery list before shopping, can help sharpen recall skills over time.

Mindfulness Meditation (Your Brain's Version of "Vacation Mode")

Meditation often sounds like one of those things you'll "get around to eventually," but hear me out—it's life-changing for building resilience. Just five to ten minutes a day of focusing on your breath (and gently nudging your thoughts back when they wander) is enough to reduce stress and improve concentration. For beginners, try "box breathing" where you inhale, hold, exhale, and hold each for four counts. It's like hitting the mental reset button. Plus, meditation helps cultivate mindfulness, making it easier to face challenges with a calm, clear mind (even the dreaded mid-week meetings).

Gratitude Journaling (Because a Grateful Heart is a Resilient Heart)

It may sound simple but writing down three things you're grateful for each day rewires your brain toward positivity and resilience. It doesn't have to be grand: a great cup of coffee, a funny movie, or the way your cat tries to help with your laptop. Over time, this habit builds emotional resilience and helps you focus on the brighter side of life. If writing isn't your thing, think of it as "mental post-its." Just take a moment to pause and savor the little things that make you smile.

Mindful Walking (A Stroll with Your Inner Zen Master)

Imagine going for a walk and experiencing each step like a mini-meditation. Try paying close attention to the sensation of your feet on the ground, the feel of the breeze, and the sounds around you. This grounding practice can be done anywhere, from a forest trail to a city block. It's a calming way to connect with the world around you, grounding your mind and relieving stress. Walking becomes a mini mental vacation—and the only equipment you need is your own two feet!

Visualization (Where Your Mind Gets to Paint a Masterpiece)

Think of visualization as guided daydreaming. Close your eyes and transport yourself to a calm, serene place. Picture the details—the sounds of the ocean, the warmth of the sun, or the feel of cool grass. Visualization isn't just an escape; it's a scientifically-backed practice that reduces anxiety and helps your brain stay resilient in the face of stress. In a pinch, you can even use it at work: imagine your desk as a beach cabana (without the sand) and feel the instant mental vacation.

Laughter Yoga (Yes, It's Real and Surprisingly Fun!)

Forget the downward dog for a minute and try a different kind of yoga—laughter yoga! It's a simple yet powerful practice where you get together with others and simply... laugh. This intentional laughter can help reduce stress, boost resilience, and bring a smile to your face. Studies show that laughing releases endorphins and reduces cortisol, the stress hormone (27). Don't worry about looking silly, that's half the fun! Whether it's laughing alone with a funny movie or joining a laughter yoga class, this light-hearted practice is a natural stressbuster.

Practice the Art of Reframing (Turning Life's Lemons into Lemonade)

Sometimes life hands us challenges that feel, well, sour. Reframing is the practice of looking at a situation from a different perspective, helping you cope better and stay resilient. Say you're stuck in traffic. Instead of stressing out, see it as "bonus time" for a podcast you've been meaning to catch up on. Over time, reframing becomes second nature, helping you meet challenges with a grin instead of a groan.

Progressive Muscle Relaxation (PMR) (A Slow-Motion Melt into Relaxation)

Progressive muscle relaxation involves tensing and then slowly releasing each muscle group in the body. Think of it as a full-body sigh of relief. Start with your toes, clench and release, then work your way up. Not only does this help reduce physical tension, but it also relaxes your mind by training it to connect deeply with your body. You'll be amazed at how much lighter you feel afterward—like shedding a heavy mental coat.

Embrace Small Wins (Every Step Counts, Even Tiny Ones!)

When building mental resilience, celebrate the small victories—no matter how small they seem! Completed a particularly hard puzzle? High five! Remembered all the groceries without a list? Cheers! Each time you acknowledge your successes, you reinforce positive behavior and build self- confidence, a core ingredient in mental resilience. Over time, these "small wins" add up, and you'll see how far you've come when facing challenges.

Practice Kindness (Because a Little Goes a Long Way)

Practicing kindness isn't just good for others, it's great for your mental health. Acts of kindness release oxytocin (the "love hormone"), which boosts your mood, reduces stress, and strengthens your social connections. It's the ultimate "pay it forward" activity, and you get the bonus of knowing you made someone else's day brighter. Challenge yourself to do one kind of thing daily, like complimenting a friend or buying a coffee for a stranger. Soon, you'll find that kindness itself becomes a natural, resilience-boosting habit.

Deep Breathing Drills (Like Hitting the Brain's Reset Button)

Simple but effective, deep breathing exercises can be done anytime you're feeling stressed or need a mental boost. Just inhale deeply for a count of four, hold for four, and exhale for four. This kind of breathing helps calm your nervous system, reduce anxiety, and bring you into the present moment. Keep it up, and you'll have an on-demand tool for resetting your mental state.

Engage in Self-Compassion (Cut Yourself Some Slack)

Finally, practicing self-compassion might be the most essential step in building resilience. Life isn't always easy, and being kind to yourself during tough times is vital. Self-compassion practices help you treat yourself with the same kindness you'd offer a friend, making it easier to bounce back from setbacks. Next time you're feeling down, talk to yourself with kindness rather than criticism. It's a small shift but one that works wonders for long-term resilience.

And there you have it! Whether you're tackling puzzles, embarking on mindful walks, or laughing your way through yoga, each of these practices builds your mental muscles and helps you find joy in the journey. So go on—play, laugh, breathe, and savor each small step toward a more resilient, fulfilled you.

Practical Advice On Managing Stress And Staying Mentally Active

Let's be real stress is practically part of the furniture in modern life, but that doesn't mean we have to let it run the show. Managing stress while staying mentally sharp isn't as hard as it sounds, especially if you approach it with a bit of humour, curiosity, and self-care. Here's your practical guide to beating stress and staying mentally spry, all while keeping your sanity (and your sense of humour) intact:

Laugh It Off—Your Brain's Favorite Exercise

Stress is a serious business, so why not laugh at it? Watching a funny movie, swapping silly memes, or trading ridiculous stories with friends can be surprisingly effective. Science backs it up: laughter lowers cortisol (a nasty stress hormone) and releases those feel-good endorphins.

Plus, it boosts your immune system, which means a good laugh is like a workout for both your brain and body—without the sweat. Try adopting a "laugh-first" policy when stress hits. Whether it's a classic sitcom, a stand-up special, or even an inside joke with friends, keep your brain refreshed and spirits high with regular doses of laughter.

Stay Connected—Friendship: The Ultimate Stress Buster

When stress creeps in, it's all too easy to retreat into solitude, but isolation is a recipe for more stress. Staying socially connected with family, friends, or even friendly neighbors can be a powerful stress reliever. Face it: venting about that long line at the coffee shop is much more satisfying with someone else! Studies show that social connections keep us resilient and mentally sharp, reducing feelings of loneliness and anxiety (28, 29). So, next time you're feeling overwhelmed, consider a coffee catch-up, a group class, or even a chat with a pet. Every interaction, big or small, can help boost your mood and reduce stress.

Move It or Lose It—The Stress-Busting Power of Exercise

Exercise is like a secret weapon against stress. Whether it's a brisk walk, a dance party in your living room, or a yoga class, movement releases endorphins (aka "happy hormones") and kicks stress to the curb. And here's a bonus: exercise is also great for cognitive function. So, while you're lunging, stretching, or grooving, you're helping your mind stay sharp as well. For an extra boost, find an activity you enjoy. It could be hiking, cycling, or even a beginner boxing class where you can pretend you're punching your stress into oblivion. Regular physical activity is one of the most effective ways to manage stress and build resilience.

Breathe Deep—Like, Really Deep

The next time life throws a curveball, stop and take a deep breath. No, really deep breathing is a powerful tool for calming your nervous system. Start with a simple technique: inhale slowly through your nose, hold it, then exhale through your mouth. Repeat a few times until you feel your shoulders drop a little. Deep breathing not only reduces stress but can also improve focus, energy, and even sleep. And if you want to get fancy, try progressive muscle relaxation, where you tense and release each muscle group as you breathe deeply. It's a little like giving your body a mental spa day.

Organize Your Life—Clutter-Free is Stress-Free

A messy space can make a messy mind. If you're feeling overwhelmed, take a moment to declutter your surroundings. Studies have shown that organized spaces help reduce anxiety and increase productivity (30). Start small: tackle one drawer or desk at a time or create a to-do list to organize your day. Set up a simple calendar to track deadlines or daily goals to give you a bit of control. An organized home or workspace doesn't just look good; it feels good too. Every step toward decluttering is a step toward a calmer, clearer mind.

Self-Care Isn't Selfish—It's Essential

When stress is high, self-care often takes a backseat. But if you're running on fumes, you're no good to anyone. Taking time for yourself isn't selfish; it's survival. Prioritize a few self-care practices that bring you peace. It could be as simple as enjoying a long bath, reading a mystery novel, or spending 20 minutes outdoors. Nature has a fantastic way of grounding us, lowering stress, and lifting our spirits. Think of self-care as a regular investment in your mental and emotional well-being. So light that candle, put on your favorite playlist, and let yourself unwind.

Screen Time Detox—Because Blue Light Is No Friend to Your Brain

Smartphones, laptops, TVs—they're everywhere, and sometimes it feels like they own us. Excessive screen time can drain your energy, disrupt your sleep, and even increase stress. Setting limits is key. Try a "digital detox" for an hour or two each day. Turn off notifications and enjoy some good old- fashioned face-to-face conversations or pick up a paper book instead of your e-reader. Your brain and eyes need a break, and they'll thank you for it. Plus, less screen time usually means more time for creative pursuits, physical activity, and real-life interactions.

Stay Curious—Keep Your Mind Engaged and Growing

A curious mind is a resilient mind. Staying mentally active doesn't have to be a chore; it can be downright fun. Pick up a hobby that you've always wanted to try, whether it's learning a new language, cooking up exotic recipes, or dabbling in DIY crafts. Studies show that mentally stimulating activities like puzzles, board games, and even reading can enhance cognitive health and lower stress levels (31). And don't forget about lifelong learning, consider taking a class, joining a book club, or even watching a documentary on a topic you're passionate about. A curious mind is always growing, keeping you, both engaged and mentally fit.

Sleep—Your Brain's Secret Weapon Against Stress

Skimping on sleep is like borrowing trouble. Lack of sleep makes stress feel bigger, muddles your thinking, and can even make you grumpier than a Monday morning without coffee. Prioritize a good night's sleep by creating a restful environment: dim the lights, keep the room cool, and ditch screens at least an hour before bed. If racing thoughts keep you up, try a simple mindfulness exercise or listen to calming music. A well-rested brain is better equipped to handle stress, stay sharp, and keep your mood on an even keel.

Practice Gratitude—Small Moments, Big Impact

Gratitude has a sneaky way of transforming stress. When life feels overwhelming, take a moment to reflect on what you're thankful for, no matter how small. Write down three things you're grateful for each day or keep a "positivity journal." Focusing on positive experiences can shift your mindset and reduce stress levels, helping you see the glass as half-full, even on tough days. It's a simple practice that not only builds resilience but also keeps your mental energy grounded in the good stuff.

Mindfulness & Meditation—Training Your Brain to Chill

Think of mindfulness as mental weightlifting. Practicing mindfulness and meditation, even for a few minutes daily, can calm the mind and reduce stress. It helps you stay present, rather than spinning out over what-ifs and worst-case scenarios. Start with short, guided meditations available on apps or online; there are options for everyone, from five-minute breathing exercises to longer relaxation sessions. With practice, mindfulness can become a go-to tool, allowing you to face life's challenges with a clearer head and a calmer heart.

Celebrate Small Wins—Building Positivity Brick by Brick

We often focus on the big picture and forget the small victories along the way. But those little wins can make a huge difference in keeping stress at bay. You completed a task early, went for a walk instead of doom-scrolling, or managed to cook a healthy meal. Celebrate these moments as they come—they remind you that progress, no matter how small, is worth recognizing. Plus, celebrating small wins boosts your motivation, resilience, and sense of achievement, helping to fuel your efforts toward a less stressful life.

Wrapping It Up: Building Your Stress-Busting Toolkit

Life's stresses aren't going anywhere, but that doesn't mean we have to let them overwhelm us. With a combination of laughter, social connections, a bit of mindfulness, and regular self-care, you can tackle stress like a pro. Remember, it's about balance: small changes, repeated consistently, can make a big difference. So, breathe, laugh, connect, and celebrate every small step—stress doesn't stand a chance. You've got this!

Importance Of Flexibility And Mobility For Maintaining Independence

Let's really dig into why flexibility and mobility are so essential for staying independent—and have some fun with it. Picture this: the freedom to crouch down to tie your shoelace without the sound effects of Rice Krispies (snap, crackle, pop) or reaching that top cabinet without needing a step stool (or a ladder…or someone taller). It's those small acts, the ones we usually take for granted, that begin to define a life lived independently. And flexibility and mobility? They're the low-key superheroes, the Clark Kent qualities, letting you stay in charge of your own life without needing to call in a squad every time you need to bend or lift.

The "Why" Behind Staying Bendy

Flexibility and mobility may sound like perks for the young, but they're actually just as essential (if not more) as we age. They're what give you the ability to tie your shoes, retrieve your keys from under the couch, or twist around in the car to make that smooth parallel park. Imagine your body as a trusty old car: flexibility is like keeping the tires well-aligned, and mobility is that engine purr that makes it run smoothly. Without them, your range of motion gets limited, and each little movement starts feeling like a strenuous task. Suddenly, the once-simple act of bending down to tie a shoelace can feel like prepping for an expedition up the Mount Everest.

But there's more to it than just convenience. When you're flexible, your muscles and joints have a natural resilience. You're less likely to strain a muscle while lifting a grocery bag or twist your ankle while stepping off a curb. Flexibility adds a shock-absorbing quality to your body. Think of it as having well-cushioned sneakers for your joints—they're ready to spring into action, taking the pressure off bones and reducing the chance of injury. Good mobility keeps your body in a state of "ready-to- go," helping you maintain a smooth gait and reduce the chances of accidental falls.

Keep Doing What You Love – No Gadget Assistance Needed

Flexibility and mobility allow you to remain active in all the ways that matter to you, minus the complicated equipment or extra assistance. Whether it's gardening, dancing, playing a friendly game of catch, or taking that afternoon hike, keeping your body limber means you don't have to shy away from the activities that bring joy and vitality to your day. And, on a practical level, it means you'll stay self-sufficient in the nitty-gritty, day-to-day tasks. Reaching the top shelf, bending over to grab a pan from the cupboard, or hauling a bag of groceries up the stairs—these can all remain comfortably in your wheelhouse without straining yourself.

Let's not underestimate the peace of mind that comes with self-sufficiency, either. When you can accomplish everyday tasks without a second thought (or a wince of pain), it gives you a sense of control over your life. And really, who doesn't want that?

Balance – The Secret Weapon Against "Oops" Moments

One of the underrated perks of keeping flexible and mobile is the balance factor. Picture this: you're rushing down the hall, phone in hand, only to step on a rogue sock. A stiff body might teeter and go down, but someone with good mobility can often catch themselves and sidestep the fall. This little advantage can make a world of difference. Falls are no joke, especially as we get older, but a body that's accustomed to regular movement is less likely to falter. Staying agile means fewer of those "oops" moments, and more of those "phew" moments, where you gracefully avoid a stumble.

Flexibility = Freedom from Stiffness

Flexibility is like maintenance for your body. Imagine you've got a rubber band that's left in a drawer for a couple of years. When you try to stretch it, it snaps—it's brittle from lack of use. Muscles and joints, unfortunately, have a similar tendency. The less we move them, the more likely they are to seize up and limit our range of motion, making even simple actions feel laborious. Stretching regularly prevents this, keeping muscles juicy and joints happy, which translates to a body that's comfortable and functional.

Just a few minutes a day can make a big difference. Think of it as doing routine checks on your own body. A little stretching in the morning, a bit of yoga or tai chi in the afternoon, these don't have to be grueling, sweat-inducing exercises. They're meant to gently maintain and nourish your body. Regular stretching sessions are your body's way of saying "thank you" for keeping it functional.

Not a Yoga Master? No Problem!

Here's the thing: you don't have to be bending yourself into a pretzel to maintain flexibility. Staying flexible doesn't mean you need to master yoga or hold challenging poses. It's more about keeping a basic, steady range of motion that allows you to move comfortably and with ease. Easy, simple stretches that you can do from your chair or while watching your favorite show can be just as effective in maintaining flexibility and mobility.

Incorporate little mobility routines that fit seamlessly into your life. Waiting for the kettle to boil? Try a few gentle shoulder rolls. Sitting at your desk for too long? Stand up, stretch your arms over your head, and feel those muscles wake up. Even little acts, when done consistently, can help keep your body ready and able to meet the demands of each day.

Future-Proofing Yourself Against Stiffness And Soreness

Imagine a world where your muscles and joints stay as nimble as they were when you were young. While time does inevitably take a toll, keeping flexibility and mobility in your routine is as close to a time machine as you can get. By staying limber, you're essentially creating a future-proof buffer against the effects of aging. You'll be better able to handle all sorts of movements without feeling stiff, sore, or out of breath.

Not only does this make life more enjoyable, but it can help save you money and time on various interventions and therapies to regain mobility that may have been lost from lack of movement.

And who wouldn't want to avoid extra visits to the doctor or physical therapist?

Independence = Living Life on Your Terms

When you stay flexible, you're essentially making a deposit into your independence bank. Those deposits build up and pay dividends over time, ensuring that you're still able to live life on your terms. Whether it's traveling, meeting up with friends, or simply being able to dress and bathe yourself without help, flexibility and mobility support you in keeping control over how you live your life.

Thus, if you'd like to maintain the freedom to live without limits, remember that keeping up with flexibility and mobility is just as important as keeping up with daily hygiene. Invest a little time each day, and your body will reward you with years of functionality and independence. It's the TLC that guarantees your independence—and, really, who can put a price on that?

So, keep stretching, keep moving, and let your body stay as flexible as your sense of humour. Here's to many years of groan-free, graceful, and independent movement!

Easy Stretching Routines And Activities Like Yoga Or Pilates

Alright, let's talk about the art of stretching. Think of it as a mini spa treatment for your muscles, only cheaper and you don't need an appointment. The beauty of these routines? They're quick, effective, and can be sneaked into your day without feeling like you've taken on a new fitness hobby. So, if you're "too busy," get ready to loosen up because these stretches can fit right into the hustle and bustle of life.

Morning Stretch Routine: Rise and Shine Like a (Less Crumpled) Human!

Picture this: It's morning, and before you've even thought about coffee, you're giving your muscles a gentle nudge to wake up. No need for complex moves—while still lying in bed, start with a full-body stretch. Reach your arms over your head, point those toes, and stretch out long. Imagine you're reaching for the stars or let's be real, the snooze button. Hold for a few deep breaths, then pull one knee to your chest, and hold, feeling the gentle release in your lower back and glutes. Switch to the other knee and finish off with some ankle circles to ease stiffness. There you go! You're already on your way to a limber day before even getting out of bed.

Neck and Shoulder Stretches: Desk Worker SOS

If you've ever found yourself hunched over your desk like a crab trying to type, you'll love these. For neck tension, sit up straight, and tilt your head to the right, ear toward your shoulder. No need to touch your shoulder—unless you're a circus contortionist, this is just about creating a stretch. Hold for 15-20 seconds, breathing deeply, then switch to the left. To add a little extra "oomph," gently place your opposite hand on the top of your head, but don't push! Follow up with some shoulder rolls: bring both shoulders up toward your ears, then roll them back and down in slow circles. Do this about five times forward and five times backward. Voila! Neck tension, begone!

The "I-Dropped-Something" Hamstring Stretch

Whether it's your pen, phone, or—let's be honest—a snack you were sneaking, every time you bend down, you can turn it into a mini hamstring stretch. Here's how: Stand up straight, and, if possible, prop one foot on a low surface, like a footstool, curb, or sturdy coffee table. With your back straight, lean forward gently until you feel a stretch in the back of your leg. This position is perfect for anyone who sits a lot, giving a much-needed wake-up call to your hamstrings. Remember to switch legs for balance. It's stretching on the go—no gym required!

Spinal Twist: Banish Stiffness and Get a Little Twist in Your Day

Here's a stretch that's both satisfying and energizing. Sit on the floor with your legs extended in front of you, then bend your right knee and place your right foot on the outside of your left thigh. Twist your torso to the right, using your left arm to brace against your bent knee for a deeper stretch. Keep your back straight and hold for a few breaths. Switch sides and repeat. This simple twist does wonders for your spine, especially if you've been sitting all day. It's like giving your spine a big "Thank you" hug!

Stretch While You Text: Wrist and Finger Magic

Thumbs sore from scrolling? Wrists stiff from typing? There's a stretch for that! Stick your arm out in front of you, palm facing up, and gently pull back on your fingers with your opposite hand. Hold for 10-15 seconds, then switch to the other hand. It's subtle, effective, and the perfect stretch for those moments when you're waiting for a reply or watching a video. Just think multitasking, but for your body!

Deskercise: Sneak in Some Seated Hip Flexor Action

Sitting is notorious for tightening up those hip flexors, but there's a fix you can do right at your desk. Sit on the edge of your chair, feet flat on the floor. Slide to one side, dropping one knee down so it hangs beside the chair. Keep your back straight and feel the stretch in the front of your hip. Hold for 20-30 seconds and repeat on the other side. This is an excellent stretch if you've been in marathon Zoom meetings and need to keep your hips from turning to stone.

Dynamic Stretches for Those Always On-the-Go

Dynamic stretches are stretches with movement, perfect for busy days. Before running errands or heading to a meeting, try a few arm circles to loosen up those shoulders, or some leg swings to get the blood flowing in your legs. Arm circles are as simple as they sound—extend your arms and make big circles, forward and backward. For leg swings, hold onto something sturdy, stand on one leg, and swing the other leg back and forth. These dynamic moves not only get your joints moving but also gently stretch your muscles, making you feel more energized and ready to take on the day.

Desk Yoga Poses (No Yoga Pants Required)

If you're at your desk, stressed, and don't want to stand up and make a scene, desk yoga is your new best friend. Try the seated twist: place one hand on the back of your chair and gently twist your upper body in that direction, breathing deeply. You can also do a seated cat-cow: place your hands on your knees, arching your back as you breathe in, and rounding your back as you breathe out. These micro-movements are like a reset button for both body and mind and can be done without any fancy gear.

Lunchtime Leg Stretch: Take Five for Your Calves

If you're running around all day or standing a lot, give your calves some love. Find a step or curb, place the ball of one foot on the edge, and slowly lower your heel until you feel a stretch in your calf. Hold for 15-20 seconds, then switch to the other foot. It's quick, subtle, and leaves your legs feeling light and limber. Bonus: you can do this stretch anywhere you find stairs, even on a lunch break or walking into the office!

Yoga or Pilates Lite: When You Have a Few Extra Minutes

Now, if you happen to find yourself with a spare 10 minutes, a bit of yoga or Pilates can be a game-changer for flexibility, strength, and calmness. Start with a few classic poses like a downward dog (for stretching your back, hamstrings, and calves) or a child's pose (a comforting stretch for your lower back). No need to go full guru mode—a few minutes here and there can make a world of difference, and you might even find that you enjoy it enough to keep coming back for more.

Quick Foot Stretches: Because Your Feet Deserve Love Too

Our feet carry us everywhere, and yet they're often the most neglected. To stretch them out, stand up and gently rock back onto your heels, lifting your toes. Then switch, lifting your heels to balance on your toes. This simple move helps stretch the arches of your feet, keeps your ankle joints mobile, and prevents stiffness. Perfect for when you're waiting in line or standing around at work!

Unleash the Inner Child with Big Stretching Movements

Finally, don't be afraid to go big occasionally! Stand up, reach as high as you can, and stretch to the sides, or do a forward bend with your knees slightly bent. Shake things out like you're a kid again. Not only does this feel good, but it releases tension in big muscle groups and gives your whole body a wake-up call. So, go ahead, get a little silly—you might find it gives you just the energy boost you need.

The Stretching Recap: It's All About Being Kind to Your Body

Remember, stretching isn't about perfect poses or timing yourself. It's about keeping your body loose, reducing stiffness, and connecting with your own physical well-being. Whether you're squeezing in stretches at your desk, while texting, or during errands, you're already doing more for your flexibility and health than you think. So, make stretching a friendly habit, it's the closest thing to an all-day spa you'll get without leaving your desk!

Tips On Incorporating Flexibility Exercises Into Daily Life

Alright, let's make flexibility our sneaky, stretchy companion through the day! If you're wondering how on earth, you're supposed to fit in flexibility exercises without clearing your schedule, let's make it easy, enjoyable, and maybe even a little quirky. Here's how you can sneak those stretches into your routine, no yoga mat or gym time required.

The "Commercial Break Stretchathon":

You're settled on the couch, ready to dive into your favorite show, when suddenly—ads. Instead of grumbling, stand up and make each commercial a mini-stretch session. Here's your guide: First ad? Stand tall and reach your arms overhead, gently leaning from side to side to stretch out your torso. Second ad? Do some gentle forward bends to loosen your hamstrings. Third ad? Grab a wall or sturdy surface and stretch out your calves. With every break, add a different stretch. By the time the show ends, you'll have notched up at least 10 minutes of good ol' stretching, all without interrupting your binge-watching ritual.

Stretch While Waiting – "Queue-Calisthenics":

Got a few extra minutes waiting in line at the coffee shop, bank, or grocery store? Turn the line into your flexibility playground. Try a few inconspicuous moves—gently shifting weight from foot to foot or standing on tiptoes to stretch your calves. Feeling bold? Sneak in some hamstring stretches by doing a subtle forward bend, as if you're "just adjusting your shoes." You might even see a smile from someone who wishes they had your stretching swagger. And if people look at you funny, no worries— they'll be doing it too once they see how limber you are!

Sneaky Desk Stretches – Your "Cubicle Pilates":

If you're chained to a desk, office stretches are a must. Start with a seated twist: place one hand on the opposite knee, look over your shoulder, and twist. Not only will your spine thank you, but this is also the perfect excuse to look around for that coffee you left somewhere. Try shoulder shrugs, wrist circles, and stretch your arms overhead to open up your chest. And for a discreet lower body stretch, extend each leg under the desk, doing little ankle circles or flexing your toes. You'll keep the blood flowing, stay limber, and keep stiffness at bay—all while your coworkers assume you're just deep in thought.

Toothbrush Balancing Act:

Two minutes brushing your teeth? You've got time to stretch! Start with a little balance challenge: stand on one foot while brushing the top teeth, then switch legs when you move to the bottom teeth. It's an easy way to sneak in ankle and leg strength. Try adding a gentle quad stretch by grabbing one ankle and pulling it toward your glutes or lean forward for a quick hamstring stretch while rinsing. Not only are you working your flexibility, but your coordination will also get a little boost—and if nothing else, you'll have a much more fun morning and evening routine!

Stretch While the Kettle Boils:

Waiting for your coffee or tea to brew? Turn this downtime into a flexibility boost. Lean forward to touch your toes or stretch out your calves against the counter. Try a few side bends while holding onto the countertop for support, or even a few lunges if you have room. By the time your tea's ready, you'll have done more for your flexibility than many people manage all day.

Bedtime Wind-Down Stretches – "Sleepy Slumber Stretches":

Stretching before bed can do wonders for both your flexibility and sleep quality. Lying in bed, try a gentle spinal twist by bringing one knee over to the opposite side while you look in the other direction—it's like saying goodnight to each vertebra. Or give the child's pose a go to relax your back and shoulders after a long day. This quiet stretching time can signal to your body that it's time to wind down, helping ease you into restful sleep while making those muscles and joints a little more limber.

Kitchen Counter Calf Raises:

The kitchen counter is the perfect height for a mini stretching session. Waiting for something to cook? Use the countertop to support yourself as you do a few calf raises, rising onto your toes and then lowering back down slowly. Throw in a few hip circles or side lunges if you're feeling fancy. It's easy, inconspicuous, and surprisingly effective. You'll be surprised how quickly a few calf raises add up, and it's a good distraction while you wait for the oven timer.

The Elevator Leg Stretch:

Elevator rides are the perfect little opportunity for a quick stretch. No one's looking? Try gently lifting each leg to stretch out your quads and hip flexors or alternate balancing on each foot for a few seconds. You can even squeeze in a few shoulder rolls to loosen up the neck and back if it's been a long day. If someone's watching, just tell them you're testing the floor's resilience—or invite them to join in!

Partner Stretching Time – "Stretch Buddies":

Have a friend, partner, or even a pet that you can stretch with? Turn it into a shared activity! Trade stretches, challenge each other with different moves, or even hold each other's hands as you both do side bends (just don't tumble over!). This makes stretching a lot more fun and can be an entertaining way to bond. If you have a dog or cat, take their lead—pets stretch intuitively all the time. Who knows? They might just be better at it than you are!

The "Stretch-to-Impress" Strategy – Social Stretches:

When you're out and about with friends or co-workers, suggest a stretch here and there. Waiting for everyone to arrive at a meeting? Start with a neck roll or shoulder stretch. The good thing about subtle stretches is that they're low-key, and who knows—you might inspire a stretch domino effect! This could make your group gatherings just a bit healthier and might even become an inside joke (bonus points if your stretch becomes a trend).

Laundry Lunges:

Doing laundry is an underrated workout, and adding stretches is an easy step to level it up. Lifting a basket? Try a squat or lunge as you set it down. Folding clothes? Throw in some hamstring stretches by reaching down to pick up each item with a straight back and a forward bend. By the time the laundry's done, you'll have stretched out your legs, back, and arms without even stepping out of the laundry room.

Stretching in the Car – "Traffic Jam Yoga":

Stuck in traffic? It's a flexibility goldmine! You can't get out of your seat, but you can still do some gentle neck rolls, shoulder shrugs, and wrist circles to keep the upper body loose. While parked, try a few seated twists by holding onto the steering wheel or the edge of the seat and gently twisting from side to side. Just remember to keep an eye on the road, of course—this one's only for stoplights and stationary moments!

The Bigger Picture: Flexibility is a Lifelong Friend

Adding stretches here and there throughout the day isn't about going full-on gymnast or mastering a yoga pose. It's about building flexibility as a way to keep our bodies moving smoothly through the ups, downs, and odd pauses of everyday life. When you sneak stretches into your day, you're not just moving more; you're building resilience, keeping joints healthy, and making it more likely that you'll move with ease for years to come. Flexibility is a lot like financial savings: a little here and there, and suddenly you've got something solid to rely on. So, go on, be that person stretching in the grocery line or lunging in the laundry room. Your future self will thank you, and who knows—you might just start a stretching revolution!

The Role Of Nutrition In Preventing Frailty

Imagine trying to drive your car across the country on an empty tank. It would sputter, cough, and eventually give up by the side of the road, leaving you in the middle of nowhere with only tumbleweeds and a questionable gas station for company. Your body, my friend, is that car, and food is the fuel that keeps it running. Especially as the years roll by, you can't just stop it off with junk and hope for the best. Nutrition isn't just about filling your belly; it's about giving your body the premium high-octane fuel it needs to keep muscles flexing, bones unbreakable, and your brain firing on all cylinders. Think of it as a daily deposit into your "anti-frailty" bank.

Nutrition: The Construction Crew for Your Body

Picture your body as a bustling construction site—it's constantly building, repairing, and upgrading. Your muscles are like cranes lifting heavy loads, your bones are the steel beams keeping everything upright, and your immune system is the security guard fending off unwanted intruders. But without the right materials (a.k.a., nutrients), this site can turn into chaos. Muscles start sagging like a deflated balloon, bones get alarmingly brittle, and your joints creak so much that you might be mistaken for a haunted house door.

The secret sauce? Protein, calcium, vitamin D, and all those good-for-you nutrients. Protein, for example, is the MVP of muscle maintenance. It's like the bricks in your body's fortress, keeping things sturdy and strong. Calcium and vitamin D, on the other hand, are the architects of your bones. Without them, you might feel like your skeleton is auditioning for a role in 'The Wizard of Oz'—you know, the one where it dances apart.

Supercharge Your Immune System

Remember that time you caught a cold and felt like a sack of potatoes for a week? A well fed immune system helps keep those moments few and far between. Good nutrition gives your body the ammunition it needs to fend off infections and illnesses. Vitamins C and E are like bodyguards for your immune cells, while zinc is the behind-the-scenes coordinator ensuring everyone knows their job. What's more, healthy eating can help you sidestep chronic conditions like heart disease, diabetes mellitus, and osteoporosis. It's like wearing a superhero cape for your insides—only instead of tights, your costume might involve snacking on blueberries and salmon.

The Anti-Inflammatory Diet: Your New Best Friend

Inflammation gets a bad rap, but it's really just your body's way of saying, "Hey, something's not right here!" Chronic inflammation, however, is like one neighbour who refuses to stop blasting music at 2 a.m.—annoying, disruptive, and harmful in the long run. Foods like leafy greens, nuts, and fatty fish can help turn down the volume, keeping inflammation in check and your body humming along smoothly.

Nutrition and Aging Gracefully

Here's a fun fact: your appetite and taste buds might start acting up as you age. Suddenly, things taste a little duller, and you might not feel as hungry as you once did. This is where "eating smarter" comes into play. It's not about piling your plate with mountains of food; it's about choosing nutrient-rich options that give you the most bang for your bite.

For example, swap out plain white bread for whole-grain options; they're like the fiber- packed gift that keeps on giving. Instead of chips, try snacking on nuts or seeds. They're crunchy, satisfying, and full of healthy fats that keep your heart ticking happily.

Protein: Not Just for Gym Bros

We need to talk about protein because it's not just for bodybuilders or people who yell "Do you even lift?" at the gym. Protein is essential for everyone, particularly as you age. It helps maintain muscle mass, which naturally declines over time. Without enough of it, you might start feeling weaker or notice it's harder to carry groceries, climb stairs, or wrestle with that stubborn pickle jar.

And no, you don't have to choke down dry chicken breasts to get your fill. Lean meats, fish, eggs, dairy, beans, lentils, and even tofu are all fantastic sources of protein. Have fun with it—make a protein-packed smoothie, whip up some black bean tacos, or treat yourself to a fancy salmon fillet.

The Hydration Station

Let's not forget about water. Staying hydrated is like oiling the gears of a machine, it keeps everything running smoothly. Dehydration can sneak up on you, leaving you feeling tired, dizzy, or even cranky (yes, "hangry" has a cousin named "drangry"). Keep a water bottle handy and sip throughout the day. Add a slice of lemon or a splash of juice if plain water feels boring.

A Balanced Plate

Creating a balanced plate doesn't have to be rocket science. A good rule of thumb is to fill half your plate with colorful fruits and veggies (think of it as an edible rainbow), a quarter with protein, and the remaining quarter with whole grains. Throw in a splash of healthy fats like olive oil or avocado, and you've got yourself a meal that's as nutritious as it is delicious.

Snack Smarter

Snacking doesn't have to be the enemy. In fact, the right snacks can keep your energy up and prevent you from overeating later. Instead of reaching for chips or cookies, try hummus with veggies, a handful of trail mix, or Greek yogurt with a drizzle of honey. These options are satisfying, nutrient- packed, and won't leave you in a sugar crash coma.

Food as Joy

Now, let's not forget that food is meant to be enjoyed. Eating isn't just about fuelling your body; it's also about celebrating life, culture, and connection. Savor your meals, try new recipes, and don't shy away from your favorite treats in moderation. After all, a life without the occasional slice of cake or scoop of ice cream is no life at all.

Closing Thoughts

Good nutrition is like a secret weapon for aging gracefully. It keeps your muscles strong, your bones unbreakable, and your immune system ready to take on whatever life throws your way. Plus, it's an excuse to enjoy delicious, wholesome meals that nourish both your body and soul. So go ahead— fuel up wisely and keep that engine running for the long haul.

Macronutrients And Micronutrients That Promote Healthy Aging

Alright, let's break this down in the most deliciously digestible way: macronutrients and micronutrients. Picture your body as a house (hopefully one with excellent insulation, a dream kitchen, and a cozy nook for reading). Macronutrients are like solid construction materials —bricks, wood, and steel—that hold everything together. Micronutrients? Oh, they're the finishing touches: the glue, screws, light fixtures, and that perfectly placed scented candle that turns your house into a home. Both are essential, and if one's missing, things start creaking—or worse, crumbling.

Macronutrients: The Big Three

Proteins – The Builders and Fixers

Proteins are your body's version of a 24/7 repair crew, complete with hard hats and tool belts. These muscle-makers don't just bulk you up like a bodybuilder; they also work behind the scenes to keep bones sturdy, immune systems strong, and tissues resilient. As you age, your body needs more protein to keep the repair process humming. It's like the plumbing in an old house—maintenance becomes a constant priority. So where do you find these little helpers? Look no further than beans, chicken, eggs, tofu, lentils, and lean meats. Imagine each meal as a construction site: a bit of protein at every meal ensures your team is always on call to patch things up.

Pro tip: Scrambled eggs for breakfast, bean salad for lunch, and grilled salmon for dinner? That's a gold-star renovation plan right there.

Carbohydrates – The Energizers

Carbs are the body's main energy source, your internal cheerleaders shouting, "You've got this!" But here's the trick—choose carbs that give you slow, steady energy, like whole grains, vegetables, and fruits. These are the good carbs that won't leave you snoozing after a mid-afternoon sugar crash.

Think of carbs as the fuel for every task you do—whether it's powering through a Sudoku puzzle or a Zumba class. Complex carbs (whole wheat bread, brown rice, quinoa) keep your blood sugar steady, and your energy sustained. Simple carbs (ahem, donuts) might taste like heaven, but they'll leave you in a foggy slump.

Pro tip: If you wouldn't put cheap gas in a Ferrari, don't put empty carbs in your body. Treat yourself like the luxury model you are.

Fats – The Unsung Heroes

Fats get a bad rap, but let's set the record straight: healthy fats are your best friends. They cushion your joints, protect your organs, and keep your brain sharper than a detective in a noir film. Plus, they're essential for absorbing vitamins A, D, E, and K.

Look for unsaturated fats, like those in avocados, nuts, seeds, olive oil, and fatty fish. These are the fats that make your heart sing and your skin glow. On the flip side, steer clear of trans fats (found in processed foods) unless you're into creaky arteries and grumpy joints.

Pro tip: Think Mediterranean diet—drizzle olive oil on your salad, snack on almonds, and enjoy a piece of dark chocolate. Yes, you read that right. Chocolate!

Micronutrients: The Tiny Titans

These little guys may not grab headlines, but they're the real MVPs of healthy aging. Think of them as the tiny nails and screws holding your house together, ensuring every system works seamlessly.

Calcium and Vitamin D – The Bone Builders

Your bones are like the foundation of your house, and calcium is the concrete. But even the strongest foundation needs help—vitamin D is like the construction foreman ensuring calcium gets where it's needed. Together, they're the dream team for preventing osteoporosis and keeping you upright.

Find calcium in dairy products, leafy greens, almonds, and fortified cereals. As for vitamin D, soak up some sunlight or add fatty fish and fortified milk to your diet.

Pro tip: If you're not a fan of milk, a handful of almonds and a stroll in the sun can work wonders. Just don't forget sunscreen—aging gracefully doesn't mean skipping UV protection!

Vitamin B12 – The Brain Booster

Vitamin B12 is like Wi-Fi for your body—essential for staying connected, energized, and functioning at full speed. As you age, your ability to absorb B12 diminishes, which is ironic because your body actually needs more of it for brain health and energy.

Where to find it? Fish, dairy, eggs, and fortified cereals are all great sources. Vegetarians and vegans might need to consider supplements or fortified options.

Pro tip: Feeling forgetful? It might not just be aging—it could be a B12 deficiency. Add a little salmon to your dinner plate and watch your memory.

Magnesium – The Chill Mineral

Magnesium is your body's stress ball, helping muscles relax, nerves function, and sleep come easier. It's like the yoga instructor of nutrients—calming, grounding, and oh-so-necessary.

Find it in leafy greens, nuts, seeds, and whole grains. If you've ever felt muscle cramps or struggled with sleep, a magnesium boost might be just what the doctor ordered.

Pro tip: A spinach salad topped with pumpkin seeds is practically a spa treatment for your insides.

Omega-3 Fatty Acids – The Peacekeepers

Inflammation is like the squeaky hinge of aging—it's annoying and potentially damaging if left unchecked. Enter omega-3 fatty acids, the natural lubricants that keep your heart strong, your brain sharp, and your joints smooth.

Find these in fatty fish (like salmon and mackerel), chia seeds, flaxseeds, and walnuts. Omega-3s are your dietary diplomats, reducing inflammation and maintaining harmony throughout your body.

Pro tip: If fish isn't your thing, a handful of walnuts or a chia-seed smoothie can still bring peace to your plate.

How To Put It All Together

Eating well doesn't mean turning your kitchen into a science lab or banishing desserts forever. It's about balance, variety, and a little bit of planning. Imagine your plate as a masterpiece: half filled with colorful veggies, a quarter with lean protein, and a quarter with whole grains. Drizzle some healthy fat on top, and voilà—you're Picasso with a fork.

Snack Smart

Skip the vending machine chips and go for nutrient-packed snacks like a handful of trail mix, a slice of cheese with whole-grain crackers, or apple slices with almond butter. These options not only taste great but also sneak in some extra protein, healthy fats, and fiber.

Hydrate, Hydrate, Hydrate

Water doesn't get the credit it deserves. Staying hydrated helps every system in your body function better, from digestion to joint health. Plus, sometimes hunger is just thirst in disguise.

By focusing on macronutrients and micronutrients, you're not just eating—you're building a resilient, energetic, and vibrant version of yourself. Think of each meal as an investment in your body's future. And remember, a little indulgence now and then isn't just okay, it's encouraged. Because what's a well-built house without a little pizzazz? Keep eating smart, living well, and aging like a fine wine—nutrient-rich and full of life.

Sample Meal Plans And Easy, Nutrient-Packed Recipes

Ah, food—a universal love language and the ultimate bridge between science and soul. When it comes to healthy aging, what you put on your plate plays a starring role in how you feel, function, and flourish. Fear not; this isn't about surviving on kale smoothies or choking down unseasoned boiled chicken. The goal is to fuel your body with meals so delicious and satisfying that you'll barely notice how nutrient-packed they are. Let's dive in, fork first.

Sample Meal Plan for a Day of Fabulous Feasting

Breakfast: Energizing Oatmeal

Why it's a winner: This bowl is your morning superhero, combining fiber, protein, and healthy fats to keep you energized and focused.

Ingredients: 1/2 cup rolled oats, 1 cup almond milk, 1/2 cup mixed berries, 1 tablespoon chia seeds, 1 tablespoon almond butter, cinnamon, and honey to taste.

Instructions: Cook the oats with almond milk. Once creamy, top with berries, chia seeds, and almond butter. Sprinkle cinnamon with the flair of a top chef, drizzle honey like an artist signing their masterpiece, and dig in.

Lunch: Power Bowl

Why it rocks: Think of this as your edible multivitamin. It's got lean protein, fiber, and a rainbow of veggies—basically, the Avengers of nutrition. Recipe:

Ingredients: 1/2 cup cooked quinoa, 1/2 cup roasted sweet potato cubes, 1/2 cup steamed broccoli, 1/4 avocado, 4 ounces grilled chicken, tahini, and lemon juice.

Instructions: Layer the quinoa, sweet potato, and broccoli in a bowl. Top with chicken slices and avocado. Drizzle with tahini, squeeze fresh lemon juice over the top, and marvel at your own culinary brilliance.

Snack: Greek Yogurt Delight

Why it works: This snack keeps you feeling full and supplies a perfect mix of protein, calcium, and healthy fats.

Ingredients: 1/2 cup Greek yogurt, 1/4 banana (sliced), 1 tablespoon chopped walnuts, 1 teaspoon honey.

Instructions: Scoop yogurt into a bowl, add banana slices, sprinkle walnuts, and drizzle honey like you're hosting a cooking show. Voila!

Dinner: Salmon with Veggie Medley

Why it shines: Packed with omega-3s, vitamins, and fiber, this meal nourishes your body and tastes so good you'll forget it's healthy.

Ingredients: 4 ounces salmon, 1/2 cup Brussels sprouts, 1/2 cup roasted carrots, and 1/2 cup cooked brown rice or sweet potato.

Instructions: Roast the Brussels sprouts and carrots with olive oil, salt, and pepper at 400°F (200°C) for 20 minutes. Bake the salmon (seasoned with lemon and herbs) for 15 minutes. Serve everything with your carb of choice and bask in your dinner triumph.

Quick and Easy Recipes for Every Occasion

Green Power Smoothie: Your on-the-go vitamin shot! Ingredients: 1 handful of spinach, 1 cup almond milk, 1 banana, 1 tablespoon chia seeds, and 1/2 cup frozen berries.

Instructions: Blend everything until smooth. Serve in a mason jar for Instagram-worthy vibes. Add a straw for drama.

Pro Tip: Freeze your spinach ahead of time to make your smoothie extra cold and refreshing.

Baked Egg Muffins: The grab-and-go breakfast you didn't know you needed.

Ingredients: 6 large eggs, 1/2 cup diced bell peppers, 1 handful of spinach, and 1/4 cup of shredded cheese.

Instructions: Preheat oven to 350°F (175°C). Whisk the eggs, then pour into a greased muffin tin. Sprinkle in peppers, spinach, and cheese. Bake for 20 minutes or until set.

Fun Twist: Add diced turkey or smoked salmon for an extra protein punch.

Chia Seed Pudding: Dessert meets breakfast in this creamy creation.

Ingredients: 1/4 cup chia seeds, 1 cup almond milk, 1 teaspoon honey or maple syrup, and fruit for topping (berries, kiwi, or banana slices work great!)

Instructions: Mix chia seeds and almond milk in a jar. Add sweetener, stir well, and let it chill overnight in the fridge. Top with fruit in the morning and enjoy the magic of pudding without guilt.

Pro Tip: For extra flavor, stir in a teaspoon of cocoa powder or vanilla extract before chilling.

Lentil and Veggie Soup: A cozy bowl of goodness, perfect for chilly evenings.

Ingredients: 1 cup lentils (any color), 4 cups of vegetable broth, 1 diced carrot, 1 diced celery stalk, 1 handful spinach, salt, pepper, and turmeric as needed.

Instructions: In a large pot, combine lentils, broth, carrot, and celery. Simmer for 30 minutes. Stir in spinach, season with salt, pepper, and turmeric, and serve warm.

Chef's Secret: Add a splash of coconut milk for a creamy twist or garnish with fresh parsley for a touch of fancy.

Some Oriental Recipes

Miso Soup with Tofu and Seaweed, good for breakfast. Ingredients: 4 cups dashi (Japanese soup stock), 3-4 tbsp miso paste, 1/2 cup of tofu cubed, 1 sheet of nori, cut into strips, and 1/4 cup of sliced scallions.

Instructions: Bring dashi to simmer in a pot. Dissolve miso paste in a small amount of dashi and add back to the pot. Add tofu and nori, simmer for 2-3 minutes. Garnish with scallions and serve hot.

Thai Chicken Salad with Peanut Dressing, easy for busy lunch.

Ingredients: 2 chicken breasts cooked and shredded, 2 cups mixed greens, 1/2 cup shredded carrots, 1/2 cup sliced cucumbers, and 1/4 cup chopped peanuts.

Peanut Dressing: 1/4 cup peanut butter, 2 tbsp soy sauce, 1 tbsp lime juice, 1 tbsp honey, and 1-2 tbsp water (to thin).

Instructions: Combine salad ingredients in a bowl. Whisk together dressing ingredients until smooth. Drizzle dressing over the salad and toss to combine.

Palak Paneer (Spinach and Cottage Cheese), suitable for dinner.

Ingredients: 250g cubed paneer, 300g spinach leaves, blanched and pureed, 2 tbsp oil, 1 tsp cumin seeds, 1 cup chopped onions, 1 tsp ginger-garlic paste, 1 cup chopped tomatoes, 1 tsp cumin powder, 1 tsp coriander powder, 1/2 tsp turmeric powder, 1/2 tsp garam masala, salt to taste, and 1/2 cup cream (optional).

Instructions: Heat oil in a pan and add cumin seeds. Once they splutter, add onions and sauté until golden brown. Add ginger-garlic paste and cook for a minute. Add tomatoes, cumin powder, coriander powder, turmeric powder, garam masala, and salt. Cook until the tomatoes are soft. Add spinach puree and mix well. Cook for 5-7 minutes. Add paneer cubes and simmer for another 5 minutes. Add cream (if using) and mix well. Serve hot with naan.

Bhuna Khichuri (Rice and Lentil Pilaf), ideal for breakfast or lunch.

Ingredients: 1 cup basmati rice, 1/2 cup split yellow moong dal (lentils), 2 tbsp oil, 1 bay leaf, 1 cinnamon stick, 2-3 cardamom pods, 1 cup chopped onions, 1 tsp ginger-garlic paste, 1 cup chopped tomatoes, 1 tsp turmeric powder, 1 tsp cumin powder, salt to taste, and 2 cups of water. Fresh coriander leaves, chopped (optional).

Instructions: Rinse rice and lentils separately and drain. Heat oil in a pan and add bay leaf, cinnamon stick, and cardamom pods. Add onions and sauté until golden brown. Add ginger-garlic paste and cook for a minute. Add tomatoes, turmeric powder, cumin powder, and salt. Cook until tomatoes are soft. Add rice and lentils, mix well, and cook for 2-3 minutes. Add water, bring to a boil, then reduce heat and simmer until rice and lentils are cooked. Garnish with coriander leaves and serve hot with egg curry.

Tips for Cooking and Eating Like a Nutritional Ninja

Batch Cooking: Make double or triple batches of soups, stews, or egg muffins. Freeze portions for busy days when cooking feels impossible.

One-Pan Wonders: Sheet pan meals (like roasted salmon and veggies) are your best friend.

Less cleanup, more eating!

Spice It Up: Don't skimp on seasonings. Turmeric, paprika, cumin, and cinnamon can transform even the simplest dishes into gourmet experiences.

Nutrient Superstars to Sprinkle into Your Meals

Seeds and Nuts: Flaxseeds, chia seeds, and almonds add crunch, fiber, and healthy fats to almost anything.

Herbs: Fresh parsley, cilantro, or basil can brighten up any dish, taking it from drab to fab in seconds.

Citrus: A squeeze of lemon or lime can elevate soups, salads, and even grilled proteins to a whole new level of zing.

Eating for Joy and Longevity

Let's face it, life's too short for bland food. Healthy eating doesn't mean sacrificing flavor or spending hours in the kitchen. It's about finding what works for you, sneaking in those nutrients where you can, and savouring every bite along the way. After all, eating isn't just about survival—it's about thriving, one delicious forkful at a time.

Sleep For Physical And Mental Resilience

Sleep is the unsung hero of health and well-being. It's the original, time-tested "reboot" button, where we hit pause on the chaos of life and allow our bodies to quietly go into repair mode. Forget Silicon Valley start-ups; the real innovation is happening while you're nestled under your duvet. This nightly shutdown isn't just about zoning out, it's when your body kicks into full-on maintenance mode. From brain detox to immune system upgrades, sleep is your in-house wellness retreat, totally free of charge (well, apart from the fancy mattress you splurged on).

The Magic Behind the Zzz's

Let's demystify sleep for a second. While you're dreaming about winning arguments you lost in real life, your body is busy doing heavy lifting. Picture a crack team of night-shift workers quietly fixing up your internal systems:

Brain Housekeeping

Your brain doesn't just lounge around at night, it gets to work! During sleep, cerebrospinal fluid washes away the metabolic waste your brain has accumulated during the day. Think of it as Marie Kondo tidying up your neural pathways. This nocturnal cleaning boosts clarity, creativity, and focus— so you'll actually remember why you walked into the kitchen tomorrow.

Muscle Repair and Growth

Whether you're a gym enthusiast or just carried 15 grocery bags in one trip (to avoid a second journey, obviously), your muscles need sleep to recover. Deep sleep is when the growth hormone kicks in, mending micro-tears in muscle fibers and strengthening your body for tomorrow's adventures.

Memory Mastery

Ever woken up with a brilliant idea? That's no coincidence. Sleep is when your brain organizes your day's experiences, filing the important bits into long-term memory and tossing out the junk (sorry, TikTok binge). If your mind is a library, sleep is the librarian sorting through the chaos.

Immune System Supercharge

Sleep is when your immune system dons its superhero cape. Cytokines—proteins that fight infection and inflammation—are produced in abundance while you snooze. This is why skimping on sleep can leave you vulnerable to catching that pesky office cold.

Why Sleep Matters More Than Ever

In our hustle-obsessed culture, sleep has become a badge of laziness rather than a symbol of wisdom. But let's set the record straight: sleep is not optional. It's as essential as food and water, and skipping it is like trying to drive a car on fumes. Sure, you might coast for a while, but eventually, you'll stall—and probably not in a glamorous way. Here's what quality sleep does for you:

Boosts Resilience

Life throws curveballs, and sleep helps you hit them out of the park. Well-rested people handle stress better, plain and simple. Why? Because sleep stabilizes hormones like cortisol, keeping your stress levels in check and your mood from spiralling into "drama llama" territory.

Enhances Physical Strength

Want to ace that morning run or simply survive a game of tag with your kids? Sleep fuels your physical endurance. Studies show that athletes who get enough sleep perform better, recover faster, and are less prone to injuries (32, 33). Sleep is your secret weapon, whether you're aiming for gold medals or just surviving the Monday meeting marathon.

Improves Mental Sharpness

Sleep deprivation can make you feel like you're wading through mental fog. On the flip side, a solid seven to nine hours sharpen cognitive function, enhances decision-making, and keeps you witty enough to win arguments (or at least laugh at your own jokes).

Guards Against Disease

Chronic sleep deprivation is linked to all sorts of nasty health issues—diabetes mellitus, heart disease, and even Alzheimer's. Think of sleep as the insurance policy you didn't know you needed. Plus, it's far cheaper than a lifetime of medical bills.

The Sleep Cycle: A Nightly Adventure

Not all sleep is created equal, and understanding the sleep cycle is key to unlocking its full benefits. Here's a quick tour of what happens when you drift off:

Stage 1: The Prelude

This is the lightest stage of sleep—basically, the "I'm still kind of awake" phase. Your muscles relax, your heartbeat slows, and you teeter on the edge of dreamland.

Stage 2: The Warm-Up

In this stage, your body temperature drops, and your brain waves slow. It's like your body is saying, "Alright, let's get serious about this sleep thing."

Stage 3: Deep Sleep (The MVP)

Ah, deep sleep—the golden hour of rest. This is where magic happens. Growth hormone floods your system, muscles repair, and your brain shifts into cleanup mode. If sleep were a concert, this would be the headliner.

REM Sleep: The Dream Factory

This is where the wild, technicolor dreams happen. Your brain is highly active, consolidating memories and sparking creativity. Bonus: your eyes do a funky side-to-side dance (hence Rapid Eye Movement).

How to Nail the Perfect Night's Sleep

Let's cut to the chase: How do you ensure a restful slumber? It's not as simple as hitting the pillow and hoping for the best. Here are some sleep hacks to level up your bedtime game:

Set a Sleep Schedule

Your body loves routine. Going to bed and waking up at the same time each day trains your internal clock to optimize sleep cycles. Yes, even on weekends—no snooze button benders!

Create a Sleep Sanctuary

Think of your bedroom as a sleep shrine. Keep it cool, dark, and quiet. Invest in blackout curtains, a white noise machine, or earplugs if needed. Pro tip: Ban your phone from the bedside, it's a sleep thief in disguise.

Wind Down Like a Pro

Pre-bed rituals can signal to your body that it's time to power down. Try gentle stretches, a warm bath, or reading a (not-too-thrilling) book. Avoid screens; the blue light is basically caffeine for your brain.

Watch What You Consume

Late-night pizza? A no-go. Caffeine at 5 p.m.? Think again. Stick to sleep-friendly snacks like bananas, almonds, or chamomile tea to ease your body into relaxation mode.

Get Moving (During the Day)

Regular exercise is a sleep booster but keep it early. An evening HIIT session might leave you wired when you're aiming for mellowness.

When Sleep Fails You

What about those nights when sleep plays hard to get? Your brain won't shut up, or you're tossing and turning like a rotisserie chicken. First, don't panic—stress only makes it worse. Instead:

Try a Breathing Exercise: Inhale for 4 counts, hold for 7, exhale for 8. It's like a lullaby for your nervous system.

Get Up (Briefly): If you're not asleep after 20 minutes, leave your bed. Do something calming, like reading or listening to soothing music, until you feel sleepy.

Consider Professional Help: Persistent insomnia? Don't tough it out. A sleep specialist can uncover underlying issues like sleep apnea or anxiety.

The Beauty of Naps

Lastly, let's talk about naps. These mini-sleeps can be a game-changer when done right. Keep them for a short 20 minutes max—to avoid grogginess. A well-timed nap can boost productivity, mood, and energy levels, making you a more pleasant human to be around.

The Final Word on Sleep

In the grand symphony of health, sleep is the conductor ensuring everything stays in harmony. It's not a luxury or an afterthought; it's the foundation of resilience, strength, and mental clarity. So, treat your sleep like the sacred ritual it is. Invest in good sheets, banish the late-night doom-scrolling, and relish every moment of shut-eye. Your body—and your witty, sharp-as-ever mind—will thank you.

The Effects Of Sleep Deprivation On Frailty

Picture this: you've spent the night playing mental ping-pong with your thoughts—endless to-do lists, old embarrassments, or maybe a late-night Netflix binge you just couldn't resist. Come morning, you're not just tired, you're practically a zombie staggering to the coffee machine, desperate for anything to jumpstart your brain. That groggy, brain-fogged state is your body waving a red flag: "Sleep is not optional, human!"

Sure, a rough night now and then won't send you spiralling into frailty, but chronic sleep deprivation? That's a whole other story. Let's dive deeper into what really happens when we skimp on shut-eye—and trust me, it's a tale scarier than your worst Monday morning.

The Zombie Apocalypse Inside Your Body

When you're running on fumes after too little sleep, your body enters survival mode. But here's the kicker: this "survival mode" is anything but sustainable. Sleep is like a nightly pit stop for your body, and skipping it means your systems are left sputtering on an empty tank.

Your immune system is one of the first casualties. Without adequate rest, your body struggles to produce the white blood cells needed to fight off infections. Ever noticed how you're more likely to catch a cold after a few sleepless nights? That's no coincidence. Chronic sleep deprivation is like leaving your castle unguarded—your immune system weakens, and every germ in town sees an open invitation.

And let's talk about your muscles. When you sleep, your body repairs and rebuilds muscle tissue. But when you skip sleep, that recovery process is cut short. Over time, this can lead to weaker muscles, reduced endurance, and—you guessed it—frailty. Skimping on sleep doesn't just leave you feeling sluggish; it literally eats away at your strength.

Inflammation: The Sleep Thief's Dirty Sidekick

Here's a fun fact: lack of sleep doesn't just leave you bleary-eyed; it sparks a full-on inflammatory response. Chronic inflammation is like having a low-grade fire smouldering inside your body. It damages cells, tissues, and even organs, leading to long-term wear and tear. Think of it this way: skipping sleep is like letting a bunch of toddlers loose in a room full of priceless antiques. It might not seem catastrophic at first, but give it time, and the damage adds up.

Inflammation also messes with your cardiovascular system. Sleep deprivation has been linked to higher blood pressure, increased heart rate, and a greater risk of heart disease. If your heart had a voice, it'd be saying, "Seriously? Can we get some rest around here?"

The Domino Effect: Sleep, Brain, and Balance

Sleep isn't just for the body, it's also for the brain. During deep sleep, your brain clears out waste products (yes, your brain needs a nightly cleaning crew). Skip sleep, and that waste piles up, slowing down your thought processes and making you forgetful. Have you ever blanked on someone's name or walked into a room and forgotten why you're there? Lack of sleep might be the culprit.

Even worse, chronic sleep deprivation messes with your mood. It can lead to increased anxiety, depression, and irritability. Not exactly the vibe you want to bring to family dinners or important meetings, right? Over time, poor mental health can create a vicious cycle, making it even harder to fall asleep and stay asleep.

And let's not forget balance and coordination. When you're sleep-deprived, your reaction times slow down, and your motor skills suffer. This increases your risk of falls and injuries—especially concerning as you age. Imagine walking around like a sleepy toddler learning to walk for the first time. Cute when you're two, not so much when you're 62.

Hormonal Havoc: Why Skipping Sleep Can Age You Faster

Lack of sleep is a hormonal nightmare. Your body releases less human growth hormone (HGH), which is essential for tissue repair, bone strength, and muscle mass. HGH is the fountain of youth your body produces nightly—but only if you let it.

Meanwhile, sleep deprivation ramps up cortisol (the stress hormone), and too much cortisol can wreak havoc on your body. High cortisol levels are linked to increased fat storage, reduced muscle mass, and even memory problems. Skipping sleep is like hitting the fast-forward button on the aging process—and not in a good way.

Metabolism Meltdown: Why Sleep Is Your Secret Weight-Loss Weapon

Ever wondered why you crave junk food after a sleepless night? Sleep deprivation messes with the hormones that regulate hunger. Ghrelin (the hunger hormone) goes up, while leptin (the hormone that tells you you're full) goes down. The result? You're reaching for that extra slice of pizza or double scoop of ice cream, even though your body doesn't actually need it.

Over time, this sleep-deprivation-induced overeating can lead to weight gain and increase your risk of developing diabetes mellitus. So, if you're trying to eat healthier or shed a few pounds, prioritizing sleep might just be the easiest diet hack ever.

Beauty Rest: It's Not Just a Myth

The term "beauty sleep" isn't just a cliché—it's backed by science. When you sleep, your skin produces more collagen, which keeps it looking plump and wrinkle-free. Sleep deprivation, on the other hand, leads to dull skin, dark circles, and even breakouts. In other words, if you're aiming for a radiant glow, eight hours of shut-eye is your best-kept beauty secret.

Sleep Like a Pro: Tips to Prioritize Rest

Feeling convicted yet? Good. Now let's talk about solutions. Here are some tips to help you reclaim your sleep:

Stick to a Schedule: Go to bed and wake up at the same time every day, even on weekends. Your body loves consistency.

Create a Wind-Down Routine: Dim the lights, put away your phone, and relax with a book or calming music before bed.

Limit Caffeine and Alcohol: Both can interfere with your sleep cycle. If you need that coffee fix, stick to mornings.

Exercise Regularly: Regular physical activity can help you fall asleep faster and enjoy deeper sleep. Just avoid intense workouts close to bedtime.

Optimize Your Sleep Environment: Keep your bedroom cool, dark, and quiet. Invest in a good mattress and pillows, it's worth it.

Say No to Late-Night Netflix Marathons: Easier said than done, but your body will thank you.

In Brief: Rest to Stay Resilient

Skipping sleep might feel like a small sacrifice to get more done, but the long-term consequences are no joke. From weakened muscles and increased inflammation to slower reaction times and a cranky mood, sleep deprivation is a fast track to frailty—and nobody's got time for that. So, the next time you're tempted to burn the midnight oil, remember this: sleep isn't just a luxury; it's a non-negotiable part of staying strong, sharp, and resilient. Embrace your inner sleep enthusiast and wake up ready to conquer the world—preferably without the zombie shuffle.

Dreamland Delights – Practical Tips For Better Sleep Hygiene

We all know that getting enough sleep is necessary, but for many, it's like chasing a mythical unicorn. One night you're out like a light, and the next you're staring at the ceiling replaying that awkward conversation from 10 years ago. If you've been on this sleepless rollercoaster, it's time to step up your "sleep hygiene" game. Let's dive deep (and have some fun) with these practical tips to transform your bedtime into a nightly dream retreat.

Set a Bedtime Routine (Your Brain Loves Structure)

Your brain is like that over-scheduled PTA mom—it thrives on predictability. By sticking to a consistent bedtime and wake-up time, you're essentially setting your body's internal clock. Even weekends aren't an excuse to break this habit (sorry, Saturday sleep-ins). Think of it like training a puppy—routine equals results.

Kick off your wind-down ritual with activities that scream relaxation. Reading a book? Yes. Watching a murder mystery? Probably not. Stretching or listening to calming music are solid choices too. And no, scrolling through TikTok doesn't count as a calming ritual (more on that in a minute).

Limit Screen Time Before Bed (Goodbye, Doomscrolling)

We've all said it: "Just one more episode." Fast-forward three hours, and now you're emotionally invested in a fictional character's love life while your circadian rhythm is waving a white flag. The culprit? Blue light. This sneaky wavelength tricks your brain into thinking it's high noon, sabotaging your body's melatonin production, the hormone that tells you it's sleepy time.

To break the cycle, aim to ditch screens at least an hour before bed. Swap your phone for a paperback or try journaling. Need a compromise? Blue-light-blocking glasses are your new best friend. They let you doomscroll in peace… kind of.

Watch What You Eat and Drink (Your Stomach Has Feelings, Too)

If late-night pizza binges are your thing, we need to talk. Heavy meals, caffeine, and alcohol are the trifecta of terrible sleep. Sure, that coffee at 4 PM seemed harmless, but it's probably the reason you're wide awake at 2 AM regretting your life choices.

Instead, aim to finish eating at least three hours before bed. If you must snack, opt for light, sleep-friendly options like a banana (hello, magnesium!) or some almonds. As for booze, it might make you sleepy but trust us—it's a false friend. Alcohol messes with REM sleep, leaving you groggy and anything but rested.

Create a Sleep Sanctuary (Channel Your Inner Spa Designer)

Your bedroom isn't just a room; it's your sleep temple. Keep it cool, dark, and quiet to give your body all the sleepy vibes. Think blackout curtains, white noise machines, and a diffuser with a touch of lavender (because who doesn't love pretending, they're at a luxury retreat?).

Ban clutter like it's your arch-nemesis. That pile of laundry isn't just unsightly, it's mentally exhausting. And for the love of all things cozy, invest in a good mattress and pillows. You spend a third of your life in bed, so don't skimp on comfort.

Get Moving, but Time It Right (No Midnight Jump Squats)

Exercise is like a magical sleep potion—but only if you use it wisely. A morning jog or afternoon yoga class can do wonders for your sleep quality. But hitting the gym at 9 PM? That's a recipe for disaster. Even light evening workouts, like stretching or a calming walk, are better choices if you need some movement. Just remember: your goal is to wind down, not hype up.

Limit Naps to Power Lengths (Because Less Is More)

Ah, naps. Those blissful midday escapes. While a quick 20–30-minute nap can recharge your brain and boost your mood, anything longer can backfire. Oversleeping during the day confuses your body, making it harder to doze off when bedtime rolls around.

If you absolutely must nap, set an alarm and keep it short. And avoid napping too late in the day, your future nighttime self will thank you.

Manage Stress Before Bed (Relaxation > Ruminating)

There's nothing like crawling into bed only to have your brain remind you of every embarrassing thing you've ever done. Sound familiar? Stress is the ultimate sleep killer, but fortunately, there are ways to combat it.

Before bed, try relaxation techniques like deep breathing, guided meditation, or progressive muscle relaxation. Apps like Calm and Headspace can walk you through these methods if you need some help. Writing down tomorrow's to-do list is another great way to declutter your brain and keep those worries at bay.

Let There Be (Less) Light (Melatonin Needs Darkness)

Light exposure plays a massive role in regulating your sleep-wake cycle. During the day, get as much natural light as possible to keep your internal clock on track. Think about sunny walks, open blinds, or a desk near a window.

Come evening, dim those lights and let your body know it's time to wind down. If streetlights or early morning sunshine are wreaking havoc on your slumber, invest in blackout curtains. And if your partner insists on reading late into the night, a good eye mask can work wonders.

Reserve Your Bed for Sleep (and the Other S-Word)

Your bed should be a sacred space for sleep. (And yes, the other S-word. We'll let you fill in the blanks.) No laptops, no Netflix binges, no awkward Zoom meetings.

If you find yourself lying awake for more than 20 minutes, resist the urge to toss and turn. Instead, get up, do something relaxing (no screens!), and return to bed when you feel truly sleepy. Training your brain to associate your bed with rest is the ultimate power move.

Be Patient with Yourself (Rome Wasn't Built in a Night)

If you've been struggling with sleep for a while, it's going to take time to adjust. Be kind to yourself. Adopting good sleep hygiene isn't about perfection; it's about progress.

Start small. Tonight, you commit to ditching screens 30 minutes earlier, or you finally swap your ancient pillow for a better one. These small steps add up, and before you know it, you'll be snoozing like a pro.

Bonus: When All Else Fails, Seek Help

Sometimes, even the best sleep hygiene practices can't overcome deeper issues. Chronic insomnia or other sleep disorders may require a chat with a healthcare professional. Don't hesitate to seek advice—your sleep (and sanity) is worth it.

Sweet Dreams Are Made of These

Improving your sleep is the ultimate self-care move. Not only will you feel more energized and focused, but you'll also be building resilience, reducing stress, and boosting your overall health. So go ahead, treat bedtime like the sacred ritual it deserves to be. With a few tweaks to your habits and environment, you'll be well on your way to nights filled with deep, restorative sleep —and mornings where you wake up ready to conquer the world.

Cardio – The Heartbeat Of Strength And Stamina

If muscles are the engine, the heart is undoubtedly the fuel pump—the unsung hero working tirelessly behind the scenes to keep your body running like a well-oiled machine. And just like a pump, when it's strong and efficient, everything else hums smoothly. But let's not get too technical— cardio is not just about heart health; it's your ticket to more energy, endurance, and, yes, a few guilt- free indulgences because you 'earned' that slice of cake after your morning jog.

Your Heart: CEO of the Body's Delivery Service

Imagine your heart as the CEO of a global logistics empire—Amazon, FedEx, and DHL all rolled into one. It's a primary job? Delivering oxygen-rich blood and nutrients to every corner of your body. When the heart's in great shape, it's like a super-efficient courier service. There are no delays, no lost packages, and every cell gets exactly what it needs, precisely when it needs it. Your muscles, organs, and even your brain rely on this steady flow of goodies to stay sharp, strong, and, well, alive.

When your cardiovascular system is in top condition, your cells practically sing with joy. Think of each pump of your heart as a love note to your body, reminding it that you care. A fit heart pumps more blood with less effort, which means you're not only surviving; you're thriving. And what does that mean for you? More energy for the things you love—whether it's hiking, dancing, or chasing after your grandkids as they gleefully test your endurance levels.

From Wheezy to Wow: The Cardio Comeback

Cardio fitness transforms your life in ways you might not expect. Remember that time you tried to climb a flight of stairs, only to reach the top gasping like a fish out of water? Or how about the last time you got roped into a "fun" game of tag and immediately regretted all your life choices? Cardiovascular exercise can turn those wheezy moments into "wow" moments. With a stronger heart, you'll power through those stairs with ease and be ready for that surprise family relay race. Heck, you might even 'win'.

The beauty of cardio is in its simplicity. You don't need fancy equipment, expensive gym memberships, or even much space. Walking briskly, dancing like nobody's watching, or taking the dog for a jog counts. In fact, your dog is hoping for this exact scenario—nothing says "good cardio" like a game of fetch that lasts longer than three throws.

Endurance: The Secret Sauce of Staying Power

Cardio doesn't just build strength, it builds stamina. And stamina is your secret weapon for handling life's little surprises. An impromptu hike? You're ready. A dance-off at a wedding?

You've got moves for days. A grocery bag that suddenly feels like it's filled with bricks? No problem. Cardiovascular fitness equips you with energy reserves to not only survive these moments but dominate them.

What's more, cardio helps regulate your energy levels, leaving you less prone to those dreaded mid-afternoon slumps. Your colleagues might wonder what your secret is when you're still perky at 3 PM while they're glued to their third cup of coffee. Just smile knowingly—it's the cardio magic.

Your Heart: The Resilient Powerhouse

Let's take a moment to appreciate how amazing your heart really is. It beats approximately 100,000 times a day, pumping 2,000 gallons of blood. That's the equivalent of filling up a small swimming pool daily. With cardio training, your heart becomes even more efficient. Instead of furiously pounding away to get the job done, a well-trained heart can take its time, pumping more blood with each beat. It's the difference between working smarter and working harder.

This efficiency isn't just about feeling good during exercise, it's about feeling great all the time. A fit heart can recover more quickly from stress, whether that's the stress of physical activity or the stress of, say, accidentally sending a text meant for your friend to your boss. (Cardio may not fix your texting mistakes, but it'll help you recover from the embarrassment a little faster.)

The Fountain of Youth in a Jog Around the Block

Cardio is like a time machine for your body. Studies show that regular cardiovascular exercise not only adds years to your life but also improves the quality of those years (34, 35). It's the difference between simply existing and 'living'. When your heart is strong, it supports your entire body in staying active, mobile, and resilient, even as you age.

Think of cardio as the anti-frailty elixir. Frailty thrives on inactivity and weak circulation. A strong cardiovascular system counteracts that by keeping your body's "supply chain" running smoothly. This means fewer falls, better balance, and a greater ability to bounce back from illnesses or injuries.

The Joy of Movement

One of the best things about cardio? It's fun! Whether it's a leisurely bike ride, a spirited Zumba class, or even an enthusiastic game of hopscotch with the neighborhood kids, cardio comes in many forms. You don't have to slog through endless miles on a treadmill unless that's your thing. The key is finding an activity that makes your heart—and your face—smile.

Plus, cardio is one of the best stress busters out there. When you move, your body releases endorphins, those magical "feel-good" chemicals that can turn a bad day into a great one. Feeling stressed? Go for a brisk walk. By the time you're back, the world won't seem so overwhelming, and your heart will thank you for the extra attention.

Everyday Wins, Thanks to Cardio

Cardio isn't just about the grand gestures—running marathons, scaling mountains, or cycling across Europe. It's also about the little wins: carrying groceries without breaking a sweat, keeping up with your kids or grandkids, and being the last one standing at a family reunion dance party. These small victories add to a big difference in your overall quality of life.

And let's not forget about the long game. Cardiovascular fitness reduces your risk of chronic diseases like heart disease, diabetes mellitus, and hypertension. It's like an insurance policy for your health—only instead of paying premiums, you're racking up miles on your morning jog or evening swim.

Wrapping It Up: Keep That Heart Pumping

So, what's the takeaway? Cardio is more than just exercise, it's an investment in your future. A strong, efficient heart keeps you energized, resilient, and ready for whatever life throws your way. It's not just about living longer; it's about living better.

Whether you're strutting on a treadmill, busting moves on a dance floor, or chasing a runaway puppy, every beat of your heart is a reminder of your body's incredible capacity for strength and endurance. Keep it pumping, and the rewards will follow—a life full of energy, vitality, and those "wow" moments that make it all worthwhile.

Cardio Fun – Activities For Every Age And Stage

Cardio has an image problem. It's been misrepresented, maligned, and reduced to a cliché of endless treadmill drudgery, sweat-soaked T-shirts, and that one guy in the gym who's always sprinting like he's late for a spaceship. But the truth? Cardio isn't just about the machines, the miles, or even the monotony. It's about joy, movement, and creativity. Think of it as an invitation to play—an excuse to move your body in ways that make your heart sing (and beat a little faster). Let's explore a carnival of cardio activities for every age and stage, guaranteed to put the "fun" back in functional fitness.

Dancing Like No One's Watching

If there's a cardio king, it's dancing. And guess what? You don't need a partner, rhythm, or even coordination, just the willingness to move. Whether you're moonwalking to Michael Jackson in your socks or swaying awkwardly at a wedding, every shimmy counts.

Why It Works: Dancing is a dynamic cardio workout that activates your entire body,

engages your core and improves balance—all while letting you laugh at yourself.

The Playlist Strategy: Craft your own cardio dance party. Choose tracks that make you

involuntarily bop, like Beyoncé's 'Single Ladies' or ABBA's 'Dancing Queen'.

Bonus Tip: For the socially inclined, dance classes like salsa, ballroom, or even hip-hop

offer a chance to learn slick moves 'and' sneak in a workout.

Walking: The Underdog Hero

Walking might not sound glamorous, but don't be fooled—this simple activity is the unsung hero of cardio. It's like that friend who never cancels plans and always brings snacks: reliable, flexible, and low-pressure.

Step It Up: Add speed intervals or incline challenges. Try walking briskly for a minute, then slow down for two. Repeat until you feel like a walking champion.

Adventure Awaits: Mix it up with themed walks—birdwatching, photography strolls, or even treasure hunts with your kids (or yourself).

Gadget Goodies: Pedometers, step counters, or fancy apps make walking feel like a mission. Who doesn't want to see their steps turn into virtual rewards?

Swimming: The Weightless Wonder

Imagine gliding through water, feeling like a sleek, buoyant sea creature. Swimming is cardio without gravity's grumpiness. Plus, it cools you off as you work up a sweat—if that's not a win-win, what is?

Lap It Up: If you're competitive, count laps or time your sprints. Not into speed? Float and paddle like you're auditioning for a mermaid role.

Aqua Aerobics: Join a water aerobics class for a splashy take on traditional workouts. These classes are surprisingly intense and endlessly entertaining.

The Kiddie Pool Cardio: Even wading and playing in water counts. Channel your inner kid and splash around for the sheer joy of it.

Cycling: Spin to Win

There's something freeing about hopping on a bike and feeling the wind in your face (even if it's just a fan in your living room during a spin class). Cycling blends cardio with adventure, scenery, and the thrill of speed.

Outdoor Bliss: Explore trails, parks, or even urban areas. Bonus: It doubles as sightseeing!

Indoor Power: Spin classes are like a party on wheels, complete with pulsating music, neon lights, and an instructor yelling motivational slogans.

Pro Tip: Consider a tandem bike ride with a friend or family member. It's twice the fun and half the pedalling effort (if you let them do most of the work).

Hiking: Nature's Treadmill

Hiking combines cardio with the magic of the great outdoors. It's basically walking's cooler, more adventurous sibling.

Trail Smarts: Start easy and work your way up to more challenging trails with inclines and rocky terrain. Every hill is a mini cardio celebration.

Scenic Bonus: The views make it worth the effort. There's nothing like a mountaintop selfie to commemorate your cardio conquests.

Buddy System: Hike with friends, dogs, or even a group of strangers (because nothing bonds people like sweating on a mountain).

Group Dance and Fitness Classes

From Zumba to Jazzercise, these classes are like dance-offs meets boot camps. They're high-energy, community-focused, and unapologetically fun.

Zumba Zest: Dance-based cardio workouts that feel like a nightclub, minus the overpriced drinks.

Cardio Kickboxing: For those who prefer punching and kicking their way to fitness (in the air, not at others).

Retro Throwback: Jazzercise is back, baby! Neon leggings optional but encouraged.

Gardening: Nature's Sneaky Workout

Gardening is cardio in disguise. While you're planting tomatoes or pulling weeds, you're actually engaging in dynamic movement and burning calories.

Shovel Power: Digging and planting? That's resistance training right there.

Squat Goals: All that bending and standing builds leg strength. (Who needs a gym?)

Harvest Happiness: Nothing beats the joy of picking your own veggies—except the fresh salsa you'll make afterward.

Playing With Pets

Got a dog? Congratulations, you have a built-in cardio buddy. Fetch, tug-of-war, or simply chasing them around the yard can get your heart racing in the best way.

Fetch Fitness: Throw a ball or stick and race your pup to retrieve it. (Spoiler: You'll lose, but your heart will thank you.)

Obstacle Course: Set up a mini agility course for your pet—and join in for double the fun.

Cat Cardio: Laser pointer + cat = surprisingly intense cardio if you chase the dot, too.

Sports: The Ultimate Cardio Combo

Pick up a racket, grab a ball, or find a frisbee. Sports are cardio wrapped in camaraderie, competition, and good vibes.

Tennis Tactics: Singles for intensity, doubles for laughs. Either way, you're chasing that ball and your fitness goals.

Basketball Basics: Shooting hoops or playing a pickup game is cardio gold.

Ultimate Frisbee: It's like tag, sprinting, and catching rolled into one ridiculously fun activity.

Everyday Activities With a Cardio Twist

Who says cardio has to look like exercise? Sneak it into your daily routine:

Shopping Spree Sprint: Power-walk through the mall (those sales aren't going to shop themselves).

Housework Hustle: Vacuuming and mopping with vigor? That's cardio and a clean house in one.

Dance Breaks: Have a mini boogie session during TV commercials or cooking downtime.

Final Thoughts: Move Your Way to Joy

Cardio doesn't have to be serious, boring, or intimidating. It's about finding what moves you—literally and figuratively. Whether you're dancing in your living room, hiking to new heights, or just chasing your dog, every little bit adds up. So, lace up those sneakers, crank up your favorite playlist, and rediscover the joy of movement. Your heart (and your funny bone) will thank you.

Cardio Health To Reduce Frailty And Other Benefits

What if I told you that cardio is not just exercise but a full-blown life upgrade? Imagine your heart and brain as two superstar teammates, high-fiving their way to a championship called 'Aging Gracefully'. And the best part? The secret to their success is as simple as moving your body. Whether it's walking, dancing, cycling, or even chasing your dog who just stole your sock, cardio is your golden ticket to staying strong, sharp, and happy.

The Heart of the Matter: Why Cardio Matters for Aging

Your heart is more than just a muscle that goes 'thump-thump'; it's the CEO of your circulatory system, ensuring oxygen and nutrients get delivered to every nook and cranny of your body. As we age, the heart needs a bit more encouragement to stay at the top of its game. Enter cardio —the ultimate heart whisperer. Think of your heart like a car engine. If you leave it idle for too long, it rusts; but take it out for regular drives, and it purrs like a kitten. Cardio ensures your heart stays efficient, pumping blood with less effort, which is critical for reducing frailty. Studies show that consistent aerobic exercise helps lower resting heart rate, improve cardiac output, and even reduce the risk of heart disease by up to 50% (36, 37). It's like giving your heart a spa day every time you exercise.

Cardio's Frailty Shield: Why Muscles Love a Good Sweat

Now let's talk muscles. Over time, we lose about 3-5% of muscle mass per decade after 30. That sounds scary, but cardio swoops like a superhero, slowing down this decline. By getting your heart pumping, you're simultaneously engaging major muscle groups, keeping them strong, flexible, and ready for action.

Here's the deal: cardio isn't just for runners or gym enthusiasts. Even low-impact activities like brisk walking, swimming, or dancing can combat sarcopenia (that term for loss of muscle mass, strength, and function). Cardio strengthens the leg muscles that keep you steady, the core muscles that stabilize your balance, and even the arm muscles that help you lift that glorious cup of morning coffee. A strong body is a frailty-proof body, and cardio is the key to unlocking it.

Brain Gains: How Cardio Keeps You Sharp

Now let's move upstairs to the brain. Cardio is like a fountain of youth for your gray matter. Every time you break a sweat, you're boosting blood flow to the brain, delivering oxygen and nutrients with express lane efficiency. This increased circulation encourages the growth of new neurons and strengthens existing connections. It's like spring cleaning for your brain—clearing out the cobwebs and making room for fresh ideas and memories.

Scientific research supports this with gusto. Cardio can reduce the risk of Alzheimer's by up to

45%, improve executive function (like decision-making and multi-tasking), and even enhance memory retention. Ever walked into a room and forgotten why you were there? Regular cardio can help make those moments a thing of the past—or at least happen less frequently.

Mood Boosting and Stress Busting: Cardio's Hidden Superpowers

Have you ever finished a workout and felt like you could conquer the world? That's your brain on endorphins, the magical mood-boosting chemicals released during cardio. But it's not just endorphins at play—cardio also lowers cortisol levels, your body's stress hormone. It's like telling your anxious brain, "Hey, chill out, we've got this." Regular cardio has also been shown to reduce symptoms of depression and anxiety. Think of it as therapy in motion—a chance to zone out, tune in, or simply enjoy the rhythm of your footsteps. And the benefits don't stop there: cardio can also regulate sleep cycles, making it easier to fall asleep and stay asleep. A good night's rest? That's just the cherry on top of your cardio sundae.

Cardio and Blood Sugar: A Sweet Solution

Managing blood sugar levels becomes increasingly important as we age, and cardio is a natural way to keep those numbers in check. Every time you engage in aerobic activity, your muscles use glucose as fuel, effectively lowering blood sugar levels and improving insulin sensitivity. It's like giving your body a tune-up, ensuring everything runs smoothly.

For people at risk of diabetes mellitus or already managing the condition, cardio is a game-changer. It can reduce HbA1c levels (a long-term marker of blood sugar control) and lower the risk of diabetes mellitus-related complications. So, whether you're dancing in your living room or strolling through the park, your pancreas is quietly applauding.

Cardio in Action: Practical Tips for Every Level

Let's be real starting a cardio routine can feel daunting, but it doesn't have to be. Here are some approachable, no-nonsense ways to get moving:

The Power Walk: Grab your favorite podcast or a good friend and hit the pavement. Start with 10

minutes and gradually increase.

Dance Party: Turn up the music and let loose. Whether it's salsa, hip-hop, or the cha-cha, dancing is cardio in disguise.

Swimming: Perfect for low-impact, full-body engagement. Bonus: no sweating!

Household Olympics: Vacuuming, gardening, or even chasing the cat counts as cardio. Who needs a gym?

Cycling: Hit the road or hop on a stationary bike. Cycling is joint-friendly and works wonders for leg strength.

The trick is to find an activity you love so it doesn't feel like exercise, it feels like play.

Cardio's Ripple Effect: The Big Picture

The benefits of cardio extend far beyond the workout itself. With a strong heart and sharp mind, you're better equipped to tackle life's challenges, whether that's keeping up with your grandchildren, exploring new hobbies, or traveling the world. Cardio gives you the stamina to embrace life fully, with fewer limitations and more energy.

Moreover, the social aspect of cardio can't be overlooked. Joining a walking group, attending a dance class, or simply meeting a friend for a jog makes exercise enjoyable and sustainable. Plus, laughter is an excellent sidekick to cardio—both are good for the heart!

The Grand Finale: Your Cardio Commitment

Think of cardio as the Swiss Army knife of aging well. It strengthens your heart, preserves your muscles, sharpens your brain, and uplifts your mood—all while helping you maintain independence and vitality. And the best part? It's never too late to start.

So, lace up your sneakers, dust off that bike, or cue up your favorite dance playlist. The journey to a strong heart and sharp mind begins with a single step—or a single cha-cha. Your future self is out there, healthier, happier, and filled with gratitude for the cardio you do today.

The Effect Of Chronic Stress On Body And Mind

Ah, stress—the silent, sneaky little gremlin that loves to pop up at the most inconvenient times. Whether it's work deadlines, family obligations, or the curious case of the "missing keys" (spoiler alert: they were in your hand the whole time), stress is there, lurking like that one mosquito you can never find. While a pinch of stress can light a fire under us—hello, productive adrenaline rushes! —chronic stress is a whole other beast. Imagine a smoke alarm that keeps going off for no apparent reason. Annoying, right? Now imagine it's not just annoying but also slowly setting your house on fire. That's chronic stress for you, quietly eroding both body and mind.

Your Body's "Stress: The Musical"

When stress rears its head, your body puts on quite the production. The curtains rise, and out-come cortisol and adrenaline, the lead actors in your body's fight-or-flight response. They belt out their tunes, preparing you to face the tiger—or in modern terms, your boss's emails. For short-term stressors, this is fabulous; you're alert, focused, and ready to tackle anything. But when the tiger never leaves, and those hormones keep performing night after night, the show starts to lose its appeal.

Stress and the Body: The Tug-of-War You Didn't Sign Up For

Cardiovascular Chaos

Chronic stress turns your heart into a workaholic, pumping harder and faster as if you're perpetually in a spin class. Over time, this overexertion can lead to high blood pressure, inflammation, and an increased risk of heart disease. Your arteries may start to resent this 24/7 stress concert, becoming stiffer and less responsive. If your heart had a Yelp page, it'd be leaving a one-star review for chronic stress: "Tried to keep up, but the constant pressure is too much!"

Immune System on Strike

Your immune system also takes a hit. First, cortisol is helpful, keeping inflammation in check. But when it's a permanent guest in your bloodstream, it overstays its welcome, like an overly chatty neighbour. Chronic cortisol dampens your immune response, leaving you more susceptible to colds, infections, and even slower healing from injuries. It's as if your body's defense team decided to go on a coffee break and never came back.

Digestive Disruption: Stress's Hidden Hobby

Ever noticed how stress can mess with your appetite, either making you want to eat the entire fridge or avoid food altogether? Chronic stress disrupts digestion, leading to acid reflux, ulcers, and even irritable bowel syndrome (IBS). It's a gut-punch, literally.

Bone Breakdown

Did you know stress could mess with your bones? High cortisol levels inhibit bone formation, leading to reduced bone density over time. So, not only does stress make you feel like you're carrying the weight of the world, but it also weakens the scaffolding that holds you up. Oh, the irony!

Stress and the Brain: A Love-Hate Relationship

Your Brain on Stress: A Drama in Two Acts

Imagine your brain is like a finely tuned orchestra. Chronic stress is the disruptive percussionist banging wildly on the cymbals. The amygdala (your emotional response center) goes into overdrive, shouting "Danger! Danger!" while the prefrontal cortex (your rational decision-maker) gets drowned out. The result? A brain that's more reactive than logical.

Foggy Thinking and Memory Mishaps

Remember that sharp, clear-headed version of yourself? Chronic stress can make that person feel like a distant memory. Elevated cortisol levels have a nasty habit of shrinking the hippocampus, the part of the brain responsible for memory and learning. It's like having too many tabs open on your mental browser—suddenly, everything's slower, and you can't remember why you started this mental search in the first place.

Anxiety's Uninvited Encore

Chronic stress and anxiety are besties who love to show up uninvited. When stress lingers, it primes your brain's fear center (the amygdala), making you more prone to anxiety. It's like the brain equivalent of your fire alarm becoming hypersensitive, going off when you burn toast or, worse, for no reason at all.

Decision Fatigue

Ever feel like even the simplest decisions, like choosing between pizza or pasta, feel like climbing Mount Everest? Chronic stress depletes your mental energy reserves, leaving you indecisive and drained. It's not laziness—it's your brain waving a white flag and begging for a break.

Stress: The Social Butterfly That Spreads Its Chaos

If only stress would keep its antics confined to the brain and body. But no—it has to meddle with your social life, too. Chronic stress can turn the most pleasant of humans into a grumpy, short-tempered version of themselves. This can strain relationships, which then creates more stress. It's the gift that keeps on giving!

The Long-Term Toll: Frailty, Thy Name is Stress

Left unchecked, chronic stress slowly chips away at your resilience, making you more vulnerable to frailty as you age. It's like an invisible sculptor, whittling down your strength and vitality one cortisol spike at a time. Your muscles weaken, your bones lose density, and your cognitive sharpness starts to dull. It's the slow unravelling of the physical and mental fortitude you've spent a lifetime building.

Daily Stress Management Techniques

While chronic stress can wreak havoc, the good news is you can fight back. Think of the following techniques as your superhero cape—your tools for reclaiming your calm and keeping stress at bay.

Breathe Like a Zen Master (or Just a Regular Human Who Needs a Break)

Breathing isn't just an automatic function, it's your secret weapon. The "4-7-8" technique, where you inhale for 4 seconds, hold for 7, and exhale for 8, is a Jedi mind trick for your nervous system. Bonus tip? Try pairing it with soothing music or nature sounds to amplify the relaxation vibes.

The Art of Mini-Meditation

Think of meditation as a mental power nap. You don't need a mountain retreat—your couch or even your office chair will do. Try apps like Calm or Headspace for guided sessions, or just sit quietly and imagine your stress as leaves floating down a river. Watch them drift away, and you'll feel your tension float along with them.

Move! (Even If It's Just a Wiggle)

Exercise doesn't have to mean Lycra and dumbbells. A spontaneous living room dance party or a brisk walk around the block can work wonders. Pro tip: Pair movement with something fun, like chasing your dog around or trying to mimic your favorite TikTok dance (badly).

Practice Gratitude (Yes, Even on Tough Days)

When everything feels overwhelming, gratitude is like a spotlight in the dark. Try a "gratitude jar"—write down one good thing each day on a scrap of paper, toss it in, and revisit them when stress tries to take over.

Laugh Out Loud

Need an excuse to binge-watch comedy? Laughter lowers stress hormones and gives your immune system a boost. Whether it's a stand-up special, a goofy meme, or that hilarious friend, laughter is self-care disguised as fun.

Get a Good Night's Sleep

A well-rested you is a less stressed you. Create a bedtime ritual: dim the lights, avoid screens, and even spritz some lavender on your pillow. If all else fails, try a weighted blanket—it's like a hug for your nervous system.

Tame the Technology Monster

Constant notifications can keep you in fight-or-flight mode. Schedule "tech-free" times, or designate a basket where phones go to "sleep" at night. It's amazing how peaceful the world feels without a constant 'ding'.

Engage in a Creative Hobby

Whether it's painting, knitting, or assembling a 1,000-piece jigsaw puzzle, creative activities let your mind focus on something enjoyable and tactile. Bonus: You get to feel accomplished when you finish that scarf or puzzle.

Connect with Nature

Nature isn't just pretty—it's medicine. A walk in the park, gardening, or simply sitting on your porch can lower stress hormones. And no, your houseplants don't count (but they're cute).

Ask for Help (Yes, Really)

Sometimes, managing stress means admitting you need support. Whether it's talking to a friend, a therapist, or even a pet (no judgment), reaching out lightens the load.

Final Thoughts: Stress Happens, but It Doesn't Have to Win

Chronic stress is relentless, but you're not powerless. With the right techniques, you can build resilience and face life's challenges with humour and grace. And when all else fails, remember sometimes the best stressbuster is simply saying "no" to one more obligation and "yes" to yourself.

Finding Joy – Hobbies And Activities To De-Stress And Recharge

In the relentless pursuit of a stress-free life, one thing is crystal clear: joy isn't just a perk, it's a necessity. Think of joy as your built-in stress-busting sidekick, always ready to jump in and rescue you from the jaws of anxiety. Hobbies, in turn, are the magic portals that unlock that joy, giving you a chance to breathe, recharge, and laugh (even if it's at your own attempt to paint a flower that somehow resembles a potato).

The best part about hobbies? They don't need to come with a checklist or a deadline. The only criteria: they make you smile, giggle, or at the very least, feel slightly less inclined to throw your phone out the window. Let's dive into some tried-and-true hobbies that can help you transform stress into smiles and turn frazzled days into fulfilling ones.

Gardening – A Little Dirt Therapy

There's a certain charm in digging your hands into the soil and saying, "Take that, stress!" Gardening is nature's equivalent of a tight, reassuring hug. The science backs it up—spending time with plants can lower cortisol levels, increase mindfulness, and bring a sense of accomplishment.

Imagine this: You plant a seed, and weeks later, behold—a tomato! Sure, it's the size of a marble and slightly lopsided, but it's 'your' tomato, a symbol of triumph over both nature and your own impatience. Gardening doesn't just beautify your space; it grounds you (pun intended). If space is an issue, indoor plants or herbs on your windowsill are just as rewarding. Basil, mint, or even a resilient cactus can remind you daily that life can thrive with a little care—and so can you.

Artistic Escapes – Painting, Drawing, or Coloring

For those who still mourn the loss of kindergarten's coloring corner, rejoice! Adult coloring books, abstract painting, or even doodling on sticky notes can be your ticket to a mini mental vacation. Don't let perfectionism crash the party—your art doesn't need to hang in a gallery. Whether your brushstrokes resemble a Monet masterpiece or a child's scribble after too much sugar, it's all about the process. Color outside the lines. Use outrageous hues. Draw a giraffe with wings. There's no judgment in this world of whimsy, only freedom. And if anyone questions your creation, simply declare, "It's avant-garde."

Cooking or Baking – Therapy You Can Eat

The kitchen is where stress meets its end… ideally, in a cloud of flour or the comforting aroma of freshly baked cookies. Cooking is a sensory playground where you can chop, sauté, and whisk your worries away. Want something low-pressure? Start with a family recipe that feels like a warm hug. Feeling adventurous? Try homemade pasta or a daring fusion dish. Even if it turns out as an inedible science experiment, you've gained a story and, hopefully, a laugh. Baking is another form of alchemy— watching a gooey mess transform into golden muffins is nothing short of magical. And if your creations are edible, the applause from your taste-testers (or just your own satisfied munching) is its own reward.

Reading – Escape to Another World

Books are the original time machines, capable of transporting you to Victorian mansions, alien planets, or even Hogwarts, all while you're still in pyjamas. A good book doesn't just entertain; it immerses, distracts, and soothes. Feel the pull of a mystery novel? Revel in the suspense. Prefer romance? Live vicariously through the characters' swoons and swoops. Nonfiction junkie? Dive into a topic that fascinates you and leaves stress in the dust.

Pro tip: Keep a light-hearted read on hand for the days when life feels too serious. Think of it as a brain massage—relaxing and guilt-free.

Music and Movement – Dance Like Nobody's Watching

If music soothes the savage beast, dancing annihilates it. Crank up your favorite tunes, clear a space, and let your body move in ways that defy logic or rhythm. You're not auditioning for a reality show, you're liberating yourself. Feel shy? Start with a private head-bob to your favorite song while brushing your teeth. Gradually upgrade to full-blown living-room concerts. Remember, there's no such thing as "too silly" when you're dancing with abandon. And don't underestimate singing along, even if your pitch scares the neighborhood cats. It's about joy, not Grammy nominations.

Volunteering – Giving Back Feels Good

Helping others isn't just a noble act; it's also a sneaky way to help yourself. Volunteering shifts the focus from your worries to someone else's needs, offering a profound sense of connection and purpose. Whether you're walking dogs at a shelter, tutoring kids, or distributing meals, the experience is likely to leave you smiling and fulfilled. Bonus: You might pick up a new skill or meet people who inspire you. Remember, no act of kindness is too small. Even a simple gesture, like helping a neighbour, can plant seeds of joy—for them and for you.

Puzzles and Games – Let's Play

Channel your inner child with puzzles, board games, or even video games. The focus required to solve a Sudoku or conquer a game level can effectively sweep stress out the door. No opponents? No problem! Solo games like crosswords or online quizzes are equally entertaining. And if someone challenges you to a Monopoly marathon, remember stress management doesn't extend to ruthless property acquisitions.

Nature Walks – Wander to Wonder

A stroll through the park, a hike in the woods, or even a quick lap around the block can work wonders. Nature has a knack for putting things into perspective, reminding you that life's challenges are but a blip in the grand scheme of things.

Pro tip: Leave your phone behind or at least resist the urge to check emails mid-walk. Let the sound of birdsong or the crunch of leaves beneath your feet be your soundtrack.

Crafting – Make Something, Anything

Knitting, woodworking, sewing, or building Lego castles—crafting is like meditation with tangible results. The act of creating, whether it's a scarf or a birdhouse, is inherently rewarding. Don't fret about imperfection. That slightly crooked scarf or wonky birdhouse has character. And if anyone complains? Hand them the yarn or the hammer and tell them to try their luck!

Comedy – Laughter Is Medicine

Nothing kicks stress to the curb like a hearty laugh. Watch a comedy special, revisit your favorite sitcom, or read a humorous book. Want to take it up a notch? Try a stand-up class or test your own comedy chops with a "dad joke" battle among friends. Just be warned: once you start seeing humour in everything, you might not be able to stop laughing—even at your own gardening mishaps. Stress doesn't stand a chance when joy steps in. Whether you're wielding a paintbrush, stirring a pot of soup, or busting a move to your favorite song, every moment spent doing something you love is a victory for your mental well-being. So, embrace the hobbies that light you up and give stress the cold shoulder.

Why Balance And Coordination Are Critical As We Age

Ah, balance and coordination—the unsung heroes of aging gracefully! Rarely do they get the spotlight they deserve. Most of us don't even think about them until something humbling happens, like tripping over an imaginary sidewalk crack or wobbling precariously while trying to put on a sock standing up (because sitting down is 'so last decade'). But trust me, these are the dynamic duo of your golden years, the guardians of your independence, and the keys to keeping life just a little less wobbly—literally.

The Slow but Steady Evolution of Our Inner Acrobat

Let's start with the obvious: when you're younger, balance and coordination feel effortless. You're basically a tightrope walker in disguise, hopping off curbs, leaping over puddles, and pirouetting (okay, maybe just pivoting) in the kitchen without a second thought. But as we age, subtle changes creep in—our muscles stiffen, our joints ache, and our reflexes go on a coffee break just when we need them most.

The inner ear, home to your body's finely tuned balance system, might start acting like an unreliable friend—occasionally helpful, but mostly flaking out on plans. Meanwhile, your eyesight, a critical ally for balance, begins to play tricks, making it harder to gauge depth or spot hazards. Suddenly, walking across a dimly lit room feels like a high-stakes game of Minesweeper.

And don't get me started on the feet. Those marvels of engineering, with their 26 bones and countless nerve endings, are like the Wi-Fi of your body—if they're out of sync, everything feels off. Over time, we lose some of the sensitivity in our feet, which means we're less aware of where we're stepping, leading to all kinds of misadventures.

Balance: Your Secret Weapon Against Gravity

Let's face it: gravity is undefeated. It's been pulling us down—sometimes quite literally—for our entire lives. But balance is your first line of defense. Good balance keeps you upright, steady, and out of embarrassing situations like accidentally grabbing a stranger's arm instead of a railing (they'll laugh later, I promise).

Think of balance as the foundation of all movement. Walking, climbing stairs, bending down to pick up a dropped sock—it all relies on your body's ability to stabilize itself. When your balance is off, these everyday activities become high-stakes missions. And falling? It's not just about pride; it's about safety. One tumble could mean a broken bone, a long recovery, or the dreaded "I told you to use your walker" lecture from your kids.

Coordination: The Traffic Controller of Your Limbs

While balance keeps you upright, coordination ensures your limbs play nice with each other. Imagine reaching for a cup of coffee without accidentally knocking over everything else on the table. That's coordination. It's the orchestra conductor of your body, ensuring your muscles, joints, and nervous system work in harmony.

Coordination becomes especially crucial for multitasking, like walking and talking at the same time (a surprisingly complex feat). As we age, these dual tasks can feel like a game of patting your head while rubbing your belly. But with practice, coordination can remain a trusty companion, ensuring you can navigate crowded spaces or tackle household chores without reenacting a slapstick comedy routine.

The Cost of Neglecting Balance and Coordination

Ignoring balance and coordination is like letting a houseplant go unwatered, it doesn't end well. A lack of balance training increases the risk of falls, and falls are a leading cause of injuries in older adults. But it's not just about broken bones. Losing your confidence in movement can lead to a vicious cycle: fear of falling makes you move less, which weakens your muscles, which makes falling even more likely. It's the domino effect you don't want in your life.

The Mental Boost of Physical Stability

Here's a little-known fact: balance and coordination aren't just physical skills, they're mental ones too. Keeping your body steady requires lightning-fast communication between your brain and your muscles. By practicing balance, you're essentially giving your brain a workout, boosting its ability to process information quickly and effectively.

Better yet, staying physically stable boosts your emotional stability. Confidence in your movement translates to confidence in life. Suddenly, you're saying "yes" to more adventures, whether it's a nature hike, dancing at a family wedding, or simply walking to the mailbox without fear.

How to Keep Balance and Coordination in Tip-Top Shape

The good news is that balance and coordination can be trained, like loyal dogs eager to impress. Here are some simple and fun ways to keep them sharp:

The One-Leg Stand Test: Can you stand on one leg for 30 seconds? If not, practice makes perfect. Add brushing your teeth to the mix for a two-in-one win.

Tai Chi and Yoga: These ancient practices are like a spa day for your balance system, combining gentle movements with mental focus.

Dancing: Whether it's salsa, swing, or the good ol' chicken dance, moving to music is a fantastic way to enhance coordination (and your social life).

Obstacle Courses: Who says they're just for kids? Create a mini course at home with pillows, cones, or even your grandkids' toys.

Balance Boards and Stability Balls: These tools turn any living room into a balance training arena. Bonus points if you can do it while watching your favorite show.

The Hidden Benefits of Balance Training

Working on balance isn't just about preventing falls—it has a ripple effect on your overall health. Improved balance enhances your posture, reduces joint pain, and even boosts circulation. It also complements other forms of exercise, making you stronger and more agile in everything you do. And let's not forget the joy of surprising yourself. There's something deeply satisfying about nailing a yoga pose or walking confidently on a rocky trail. It's proof that age is just a number—and you're not letting it boss you around.

The Lighter Side of Wobbles

Of course, balance training has its moments of hilarity. Ever tried a tree pose in yoga and ended up looking like a wind-blown sapling? Or attempted to navigate a crowded buffet line without toppling the dessert tower? These moments remind us that aging doesn't have to be so serious. A little laughter goes a long way in making the journey enjoyable.

So, let's give balance and coordination the standing ovation they deserve. They're not just skills; they're life preservers, confidence boosters, and the ultimate aging hacks. By keeping these abilities in shape, you're investing in your independence, your safety, and your ability to enjoy life's adventures—one steady step at a time. And hey, if you ever do trip over that invisible crack, just remember it's not the fall that defines you; it's how stylishly you recover. Keep laughing, keep practicing, and keep moving forward.

Simple Balance Exercises And Games To Boost Stability

Ready to train your inner tightrope walker? Fear not, you won't need circus skills to improve your balance!

Balance isn't just about staying upright; it's about giving your body the confidence to tackle the unexpected—be it a slippery sidewalk or a mischievous cat darting between your feet. The good news is that balance exercises are not only effective but also fun (yes, really). Think of these as mini adventures for your stability muscles, wrapped up in playful challenges. Here's an extended guide to simple balance exercises and games that will boost your stability while adding a splash of humour and joy to your day.

The Flamingo Stance: Channel Your Inner Bird

Feeling fancy? The Flamingo Stance is your go-to move. Lift one foot slightly off the ground and hold the pose like you're a flamingo surveying the marshlands (or your living room).

How to do it: Stand near a sturdy chair or countertop for safety. Lift one foot off the ground and bend your knee slightly. Hold for 30 seconds, then switch legs. Pro tips: Close your eyes for an extra challenge (just don't blame me if you wobble). Hold a yoga block or a light book overhead for added intensity.

Why it works: It strengthens your core and stabilizing muscles, turning you into a balance ninja, ready to dodge life's surprises.

Tightrope Walking (Without the Risky Tightrope)

No acrobatics required here—just a pretend line on the floor and your best heel-to-toe walking skills. This exercise sharpens coordination and balance with zero risk of plunging into the abyss.

How to do it: Imagine (or tape) a straight line on the floor. Walk slowly, placing one foot directly in front of the other, heel touching the toe. Keep your arms out like a tightrope walker for balance.

Level up: Try walking backward along the line—your brain will work overtime! Add a prop, like balancing a book on your head.

Why it works: This exercise is a trifecta of focus, coordination, and stability. Plus, it's oddly meditative!

Rock the Boat: Sway Like the Waves

Picture yourself as a boat bobbing gently on the water—calm, serene, and just a little wobbly. This movement teaches your body how to shift weight gracefully. How to do it: Stand with feet hip-width apart.

Slowly shift your weight onto one foot, lifting the opposite foot slightly off the ground. Return to the center and repeat on the other side.

Make it fun: Play ocean sounds in the background for ambiance. Pretend you're the captain of a tiny sailboat navigating stormy seas.

Why it works: This exercise engages your core, leg muscles, and ankles, all essential for daily balance.

Balloon Balance: Channel Your Inner Child

Nothing says "fun" like batting a balloon around. This deceptively simple game hones your reflexes and hand-eye coordination while keeping you light on your feet.

How to do it: Toss a balloon in the air and keep it afloat using your hands (no cheating with furniture!). Stay in place or try balancing on one leg while you play.

Challenge mode: Use just one hand. Add more balloons—two or three will turn this into a comedy routine.

Why it works: It's playful, unpredictable, and a sneaky way to work on your balance and agility. Plus, laughter is guaranteed.

One-Legged Squats: Tiny but Mighty

These mini squats pack a punch without the intimidation factor of full squats. They're all about building strength and stability in your lower body.

How to do it: Stand on one leg and bend your knee slightly to lower yourself a few inches. Return to standing and repeat 5-10 times per leg.

Spice it up: Hold onto a counter for support or go rogue and try without. Add a small weight or water bottle for resistance.

Why it works: This move targets your quadriceps, glutes, and core, creating a powerhouse of stability.

The Heel-to-Toe Challenge: Tiptoeing to Triumph

Think of this as a static version of tightrope walking. It's simple, effective, and surprisingly tricky when you add extra layers of difficulty.

How to do it: Place one foot directly in front of the other so the heel touches the toes. Hold the position for 10-15 seconds, then switch feet.

Boost the fun: Try closing your eyes. Add a balancing act, like holding a water bottle in each hand. Why it works: This exercise improves static balance and concentration.

The Dance-Off: Groove for Balance

Dancing isn't just fun—it's a fantastic way to improve balance while letting loose. Whether it's salsa, waltz, or freestyle, dancing combines rhythm and movement in the most delightful way.

How to do it: Put on your favorite upbeat song. Incorporate spins, side steps, and dips to test your balance.

Why it works: Dancing challenges your coordination, spatial awareness, and stability, all while delivering a dose of joy.

The Tree Pose: Classic Yoga Charm

This yoga staple is excellent for calming your mind and strengthening your balance.

How to do it: Stand on one leg and place the sole of the other foot against your ankle, calf, or thigh. Hold for 20-30 seconds, then switch legs.

Why it works: This pose strengthens your core, improves posture, and adds a zen vibe to your routine.

Making Balance Part of Your Day

The beauty of these exercises is their simplicity, you can do them anywhere! Sneak them into daily tasks: balance on one leg while brushing your teeth, do the Flamingo Stance while waiting for the kettle, or practice tightrope walking during TV commercials.

Balance training isn't just about stability; it's about reclaiming your confidence. So go ahead—be the flamingo, the tightrope walker, the dancer. With these exercises, you'll stay grounded (pun intended) and ready for whatever life throws your way!

How Balance Training Prevents Falls And Supports Independence

Here's the thing about gravity: it's a constant companion, but sometimes it feels like it's out to get us—especially as we age. Falls are no laughing matter, but let's not tumble into despair just yet. The solution? Balance training: the unsung hero of aging gracefully. It's not just about staying upright; it's about empowering yourself to walk through life with confidence, poise, and a sprinkle of humour. The Fall-Prevention Superpower

Think of balance training as your superhero cape. While we can't always avoid banana peels (both literal and metaphorical), a well-trained body and brain can often save the day. When your foot finds a wobbly surface—be it a loose paving stone or your grandson's rogue toy truck—good balance ensures your muscles, joints, and reflexes spring into action faster than you can say, "Oops!"

This isn't just about quick reflexes. Balance training strengthens your stabilizing muscles, those unsung champions in your core, hips, and legs. These muscles work together to keep you grounded, even when the world seems determined to make you wobble. Coordination gets an upgrade, too. No more limbs flailing like you're auditioning for a slapstick comedy—your body learns to work as a cohesive team.

Independence: The True Prize

Why does this matter? Because with better balance, you're not just surviving; you're thriving. Falling isn't just about a bruised hip; it's about the fear it instils. That fear can shrink your world — avoiding stairs, skipping outings, hesitating to play with your grandkids. But when your balance is on point, that fear shrinks instead.

Picture this: instead of tiptoeing cautiously across a gravel path, you stride confidently, even daring to look up at the scenery instead of staring at your feet. You join your family on hikes, twirl on the dance floor, and tackle a staircase without clutching the railing for dear life. Balance training unlocks a life where you 'live' more and worry less.

The Core Connection

Balance training isn't just about preventing that 'oops' moment; it's about overall physical vitality. At its heart (or rather, its 'core'), balance training strengthens the center of your body. A strong core means better posture, reduced back pain, and less strain on your joints. Suddenly, everyday activities—like carrying groceries or bending down to pick up the mail—feel like less of a chore.

And let's not overlook stamina. With improved balance and core strength, you move more efficiently, conserving energy. Whether it's gardening, chasing your grandkids, or taking the long way home for an extra stroll, you'll find yourself with the endurance to keep going.

Brain Benefits of Balance

Balance isn't just a physical skill; it's a mental workout too. Your brain plays an integral role, processing feedback from your body and surroundings to make split-second decisions. Balance training sharpens your focus and reaction time, keeping your mind as agile as your body.

Here's the kicker: practicing balance might even boost your memory. Studies suggest challenging physical activities, like balance exercises, stimulate brain regions responsible for cognition (38). So, while you're perfecting your tree pose, you're also planting seeds for mental sharpness.

Making Balance Training Fun

Let's face it: nobody wants to spend hours standing on one leg staring at a wall. The secret to sticking with balance training is finding the fun.

Dance it out: Ballroom dancing isn't just romantic; it's a killer balance workout. Salsa, tango, or even swing dancing will have you gracefully shifting your weight and keeping your stability. Bonus points for looking fabulous while at it.

Martial arts magic: Tai chi and qigong blend gentle movements with focus and balance, all while making you feel like a Zen master.

Yoga: Wobble in style: From warrior poses to balancing on one foot, yoga is the perfect mix of challenge and calm. And if you tip over? No one's judging. Yoga is all about embracing the process.

Games and gadgets: Turn balance training into playtime. Try walking heel-to-toe like you're on an invisible tightrope or invest in a wobble board and challenge your grandkids to a "who can stay up longest" contest. Spoiler: with practice, you'll win.

Real-Life Stories: Balance in Action

Need more convincing? Meet Barbara, 72. After starting a simple balance routine, she went from skipping her favorite hiking trails to conquering a rocky mountain path with her grandkids. "I feel like I've found my footing again—literally," she says with a laugh.

Then there's Joe, 68, who swears ballroom dancing. "I've fallen in love with dancing 'and' stopped falling altogether," he jokes. "My wife's thrilled about both."

The Ripple Effect

Balance training isn't just about avoiding falls; it has a ripple effect across your entire life. Improved balance means better mobility, which means staying active and socially connected. Whether it's joining a fitness class, walking your dog, or participating in community activities, balance training ensures you stay engaged and independent.

Even your wardrobe benefits! Who doesn't love the confidence to wear those slightly-too-high shoes or strut in style without worrying about a misstep?

When to Start? Yesterday!

Here's the beauty of balance training: it's never too late to start. Whether you're 40, 70, or beyond, your body is ready to learn. Start small—maybe a few minutes standing on one leg while brushing your teeth. Build from there with guided classes or exercises tailored to your fitness level. And don't worry if you wobble. In fact, embrace it. Every wobble is a tiny triumph, a sign that your body is learning and adapting. Celebrate the process, and before you know it, you'll be balancing like a pro.

Final Thoughts: Balance is the Best Gift

Balance training is like a secret handshake with your future self—a promise that you're setting them up for a life of stability, confidence, and joy. It's not just about avoiding falls; it's about stepping boldly into a world of possibilities.

So go ahead, wobble, laugh, and keep training. Every small effort you put into your balance now pays off in spades down the road. And remember life's greatest adventures often require a little daring and a lot of balance.

Role Of Social Connections In Healthy Aging And Frailty

Let's be honest: humans are social creatures. Sure, we all have days when the idea of peopleing is exhausting, but in the grand scheme of things, we thrive on connection. Whether it's the familiar warmth of a friend's smile, the ridiculous joy of an inside joke, or the simple pleasure of venting about the price of avocados, our social bonds are our lifelines.

But what if I told you these connections are more than just good vibes? That every coffee date, heartfelt conversation, and game of cards with your neighbour is actually a secret weapon in the quest for healthy aging and mental wellness? Yes, folks, being social is not just fun—it's practically medicinal. Let's unpack this with a dash of humour and a whole lot of heart.

Why Social Connections Are the Swiss Army Knife of Healthy Aging

Think of your social connections as the multitool you didn't know you needed. They tackle everything from loneliness to longevity with an effortless charm. Research consistently shows that maintaining strong social ties as we age can improve physical health, bolster mental resilience, and keep cognitive decline at bay. In other words, chatting with your bestie might actually be adding years to your life.

Here's how it works: when we engage in meaningful interactions, our brains reward us with a delightful cocktail of chemicals like dopamine and oxytocin. Oxytocin, often called the "bonding hormone," is like a warm hug for your brain, reducing stress, lowering blood pressure, and even helping your body heal faster. (No offense to kale, but I'll take oxytocin over a green smoothie any day.)

Moreover, these connections create a positive feedback loop. Feeling valued and understood motivates us to engage more, which in turn strengthens our mental health and keeps us energized. It's a cycle so rewarding, it might just beat the thrill of finding exact change at the bottom of your bag.

Social Butterflies Live Longer (and Laugh More)

Ever noticed how people with active social lives seem to carry a certain sparkle? They've got the glow of connection, and it's not just skin deep. Longevity studies reveal that individuals with robust social networks live longer than their more isolated peers (39). And we're not talking about hermit- level isolation here; even small social interactions—like chatting with the barista or waving your neighbour—add up.

One theory is that being social reduces chronic stress, a notorious villain in the aging process. Stress wears down your immune system, muddles your brain, and can leave you feeling like a grumpy cat meme come to life. Strong social bonds act like a buffer, turning major stressors into manageable speed bumps. And let's not forget the mental benefits. Sharing experiences, whether joyful or challenging, gives life meaning. It reminds us that we're not alone in this wild ride, even when things get messy. After all, misery may love company, but so does laughter, joy, and the occasional embarrassing story.

The Perils of Loneliness: A Silent Health Risk

Loneliness doesn't just feel bad, it's downright hazardous to your health. Studies equate chronic loneliness with smoking 15 cigarettes a day (40). Yes, you read that right: being socially isolated is as bad for you as chain-smoking. (Although, let's be clear, doing both is a hard pass.)

For older adults, loneliness can snowball into more serious problems. Prolonged isolation increases the risk of depression, anxiety, and cognitive decline. It's also linked to higher rates of Alzheimer's and other dementias. Without the mental stimulation and emotional comfort that social interactions provide, our brains can start to lose their edge, much like an unused kitchen knife.

But the antidote is simple: connection. Reaching out to others—even in small, mundane ways—can reverse the effects of loneliness and keep our mental gears turning. Think of it like rebooting a sluggish computer: a little interaction can go a long way in restoring function and clarity.

Connection, Confidence, and a Side of Belly Laughs

Here's the secret sauce of healthy aging: it's not just about avoiding loneliness; it's about embracing joy. Social connections provide the perfect backdrop for moments of levity, shared triumphs, and even the occasional harmless gossip session. These interactions remind us of who we are outside of the aches and pains of getting older.

Picture this: you're at a community potluck, juggling a plate of casseroles while someone cracks a joke about their third failed attempt at sourdough bread. Laughter erupts, and for a moment, everyone forgets their graying hair and creaky knees. That shared joy is what makes aging less about loss and more about resilience.

Building Bridges, Not Fences

If you're thinking this all sounds wonderful but also a tad overwhelming, fear not. Cultivating social connections doesn't mean reinventing yourself as a social butterfly. Small, consistent efforts can build a sturdy social safety net.

Start local. Chat with a neighbour, strike up a conversation at the park, or join a local club. Proximity often leads to the most enduring connections.

Combine interests with interaction. Whether it's a book club, yoga class, or gardening

group, shared activities make bonding effortless.

Embrace technology. From video calls with grandkids to online communities, the digital world offers endless opportunities for connection. (Bonus: tech-savvy grandparents are instant rockstars in the family.)

Be a little bold. Say yes to invitations, even when you'd rather stay home with your slippers.

Chances are, you'll come back feeling energized and glad you went.

When Small Gestures Make Big Differences

Don't underestimate the power of tiny acts of kindness in strengthening your social ties. A quick text to check in, a handwritten note, or a shared photo from the past can rekindle old connections and deepen existing ones. Relationships thrive on these little reminders that we care. And remember, it's not about the quantity of relationships but the quality. A handful of genuine connections can do more for your health and happiness than a roomful of acquaintances. So, focus on the people who make your soul smile.

Final Thoughts: Staying Connected for the Long Haul

As we navigate the ever-changing landscape of aging, one thing remains constant: the power of human connection. It's the thread that ties our stories together, the glue that holds us steady, and, occasionally, the reason we laugh until we cry.

So, the next time you're tempted to skip that coffee date or decline that party invitation, think again. Socializing isn't just a pastime, it's a lifeline. And who knows? That random conversation about the weather might just be the spark that keeps your mind sharp, your heart light, and your soul brimming with joy.

In the grand tapestry of life, our connections are the brightest threads. Cherish them, nurture them, and don't be afraid to weave a few more. After all, aging with grace isn't about doing it alone— it's about doing it together, one laugh, one hug, and one unforgettable moment at a time.

Ideas For Building And Maintaining A Supportive Social Network

Now that we've established just how important it is to have a robust social network (and no, I don't mean the number of "likes" on your cat photos), let's dive into the fun part: creating and nurturing a circle of supportive friends. Building relationships doesn't require the finesse of a Michelin- star chef assembling a soufflé. It's more like crafting a hearty stew—add a pinch of humour, a dollop of kindness, and a generous dash of effort, and you're well on your way.

Reach Out, Even If It's Awkward

Here's the thing about reaching out—it always feels slightly awkward at first. It's like the first dance at a wedding: everyone's a bit shy until the DJ plays something irresistible. That said, the reward far outweighs the initial discomfort.

Start small: compliment someone's outfit, ask about their dog (even if it's a squirrel on a leash— hey, conversation is conversation), or comment on the weather. A simple "How's it going?" can open doors to friendships you never expected. Sure, you might get the occasional monosyllabic reply, but for every person who gives you a blank stare, another will light up, thrilled that you made the effort. And yes, you might fumble a greeting here and there. But guess what? That's relatable! Awkwardness is the universal icebreaker. Own it. Be the person who laughs at their own mistakes. People love that.

Embrace Technology—Yes, Even If It's Confusing

We live in a world where staying connected is as easy as pressing a few buttons—or, at least, it 'looks' that way. If you've ever tried to video call and ended up staring at your own ear on the screen, you're not alone. Technology can be intimidating, but it's also a lifeline for socializing.

Start simple: text a friend, join a Facebook group for your favorite hobby, or schedule regular family calls. If you're feeling adventurous, explore apps like Meetup to find local gatherings or virtual clubs. And if you're staring at your device wondering how to set up a profile, tech workshops for beginners are not only helpful but also a great way to meet others who are navigating the same digital waters.

Social media doesn't have to be a highlight reel of brunches and vacation sunsets. Use it to send funny memes, join interest groups, or share moments that genuinely matter to you. Connection is the goal—not perfection.

Rediscover Old Friends—Your History Goldmine

Remember that friend who always saved you a seat in high school or the coworker who made endless Zoom meetings bearable? They're still out there! Reconnecting with old friends is like opening a time capsule of good vibes.

Send a message that says, "I was just thinking about the time we [insert hilarious memory here]. How are you?" You'd be amazed at how many people respond with warmth and enthusiasm. Old friends know your quirks, your sense of humour, and your history. The conversation flows naturally, and before you know it, you'll be swapping life updates and reminiscing about the time you got lost on the way to the prom.

Try a Class or Hobby Group

Let's face it: small talk can be dreadful. That's where hobby groups come in. Whether you're into knitting, pottery, or ukulele-playing, shared interests provide a built-in conversation starter.

Picture this: you show up at a beginner's yoga class. As everyone struggles to nail the "tree pose" without toppling over, there's laughter, mutual commiseration, and—voilà! —new connections. It's like team building, but without the awkward trust falls.

Many communities offer hobby classes at libraries, community centers, or online platforms. You might pick up a new skill, discover a hidden talent, or simply enjoy the camaraderie of shared curiosity.

Volunteer for a Cause You Love

Few things bond people like working together for a common cause. Volunteering is the ultimate win-win—you make a difference while meeting like-minded people.

You love animals and decide to walk dogs at a shelter. Or you have a knack for storytelling and want to read to kids at the library. Whatever your passion, there's a volunteer opportunity waiting. The shared mission creates an instant connection, and soon you'll be swapping life stories while painting a community mural or serving meals at a soup kitchen.

Be a Regular at Your Favorite Spots

Ever notice how the guy at the coffee shop who orders the same thing every day knows everyone? There's a reason for that. Frequenting the same place creates a sense of community, turning strangers into familiar faces.

Find your spot—a café, a park, a gym class—and make it a habit. Over time, you'll start to recognize regulars, and they'll recognize you. Before you know it, you'll have your own little Cheers moment ("Norm!"), where everybody knows your name.

Join a Club or Support Group

Whether you're dealing with a life challenge or just want to play cards, there's a group out there for you. Support groups and clubs are designed to foster connection. Everyone shows up for the same reason: to meet others and share experiences.

Support groups offer a safe space to open up, while clubs provide an opportunity to bond over shared interests. Both help you find your tribe, whether that's people who also love bridge or those navigating a similar health journey.

Celebrate the Little Moments

Friendship isn't built on grand gestures; it's the small, everyday moments that count. Send a quick "thinking of you" text. Share a funny article. Remember birthdays and celebrate milestones, no matter how small.

These little acts of kindness create a ripple effect. People feel valued, and they reciprocate. The more you nurture your connections, the stronger they grow.

Throw a Friendship Party

Who says parties are just for birthdays? Host a casual get-together—a potluck, a game night, or even a tea party. Invite people from different parts of your life and watch as connections bloom.

Worried about being the "host with the most"? Relax. People are there for the company, not your hors d'oeuvres. Even if you serve chips straight from the bag, your effort to bring people together will be appreciated.

Be Open to Serendipity

Sometimes, the best connections happen when you least expect them. Say yes to that neighborhood block party or the random invitation to a community event.

Be open to meeting new people, even if it feels out of your comfort zone. You never know when you might click with someone over a shared love of cheesy movies or an inside joke about the terrible coffee at the event.

Practice the Art of Listening

When building relationships, being a good listener is key. Show genuine interest in others' stories, and don't be afraid to ask follow-up questions.

People appreciate feeling heard, and active listening lays the groundwork for meaningful connections. Plus, you'll learn all kinds of fascinating titbits, like your neighbour's secret lasagna recipe or your coworker's moonlighting gig as a jazz musician.

Laugh Often and Don't Take It Too Seriously

Friendship is meant to be fun! Don't stress about having the perfect network or being the life of the party. Focus on enjoying the moments and being authentic.

Laugh at yourself, embrace the quirks of others, and cherish the connections you make along the way. At the end of the day, relationships are about shared joy, mutual support, and the occasional ridiculous inside joke.

Final Thoughts

Building and maintaining a supportive social network doesn't have to be a daunting task. It's about putting yourself out there, embracing the awkwardness, and savouring the little victories. Remember, friendships grow like plants; they need time, care, and the occasional sprinkle of humour. So go ahead, send that text, join that group, and order your "usual" with pride. Your future self—and your blossoming social circle—will thank you.

Approaches To Engage With Community Activities For Added Purpose And Joy

Ever notice how being part of something bigger than yourself feels like hitting a reset button for your soul? Engaging with community activities doesn't just add structure to your days or give you reasons to get dressed (though that's a nice perk). It fills your life with purpose, joy, and a whole lot of moments that make you say, "Well, that was unexpected!" Whether you're planting a tree with your neighbors or awkwardly attempting to dance at the local senior center, community involvement has a magic way of connecting us to others and the world around us. Let's dive into the fun, funny, and heartwarming ways to embrace this community spirit.

Attend Local Events (Even If You're Not Sure What They Are!)

From farmers markets to quirky town parades, local events are like buffets for your social life. You don't need to be an art aficionado to enjoy an art show or a veggie connoisseur to strike up a conversation at the farmers market. These gatherings are low-pressure, high-reward chances to mingle with your neighbors and soak up the lively buzz of community life.

Even if you accidentally stumble into a dog costume contest or an outdoor ukulele jam session, just go with it. Bonus points if you end up clapping along awkwardly or making small talk with someone about the weather (a classic icebreaker). It's not about fitting in; it's about showing up and enjoying the ride.

Join a Class or Workshop: From "Meh" to "Masterpiece"

There's something thrilling about learning a new skill—especially when there's no final exam involved. Community centers, libraries, and senior programs are treasure troves of classes in everything from tai chi to watercolour painting to bread baking.

Picture this: you show up to a pottery class thinking you'll make a lopsided mug, and suddenly you're channelling your inner Michelangelo. Or maybe not—but either way, you'll meet fellow enthusiasts and leave with at least one funny story about your attempts to "center the clay." And if you're not the next great artisan? Who cares? The real masterpiece is the laughter and camaraderie along the way.

Get Involved in Local Causes: Heroes Wear Gardening Gloves

Volunteering is like a secret handshake with your community. Whether you're organizing a park clean-up, joining a fundraising walk, or delivering meals to those in need, you'll connect with kindred spirits who share your passion for making the world a little brighter.

Imagine bonding with someone over a shared struggle to wrangle an unwieldy tree sapling into the ground or laughing at your inability to fold hospital corners while making a bed for shelter. These shared moments of doing good not only benefit others but also fill your heart in a way that's hard to describe—except to say it feels pretty darn great.

Become a Mentor (or Find One): Passing the Baton

Got wisdom to share? Of course you do! Mentoring is like passing the torch of experience to someone navigating the path you once walked. Whether you're guiding a young professional, helping a student with career advice, or simply lending a sympathetic ear, your insights are invaluable.

And hey, mentoring isn't a one-way street. If you're tackling something new—say, navigating the digital world or perfecting your sourdough starter—you can find a mentor of your own. Intergenerational mentoring is like a dance of knowledge: sometimes you lead, sometimes you follow, but you always come away enriched.

Visit Community Centers and Senior Spaces: Bingo and Beyond

Let's be real: community and senior centers have an unfair reputation for being stuffy or slow-paced. But step inside, and you'll find a world of energy and enthusiasm. From dance nights to trivia challenges, these spaces are hubs of connection and creativity.

Yes, there's bingo (and it's surprisingly competitive), but there's also yoga, book clubs, and even karaoke nights where you can belt out classics with gusto. Nervous about walking in for the first time? Just remember that everyone else there was once a newbie too—and they're likely more welcoming than you expect.

Participate in Faith or Spiritual Groups: Food for the Soul

If spirituality or faith is part of your life, getting involved with a local group can be profoundly fulfilling. Faith-based communities often host study groups, volunteer opportunities, and social events that help foster deep, meaningful connections.

Whether you're participating in a food drive, joining a choir, or attending a candlelit service, these activities nurture a sense of belonging and purpose. Plus, these groups tend to attract some of the most encouraging and kind-hearted people you'll ever meet. It's like a warm hug for your spirit.

Organize a Small Gathering: Social Butterflies Start Here

Don't wait for someone else to plan the fun—be the catalyst! Hosting a casual gathering doesn't have to be stressful. Invite a few neighbors for coffee, organize a board game night, or start a book club where discussing the book is optional (we all know it's more about the snacks and laughs).

These small gatherings can be the seeds of deeper friendships and regular meetups. Before you know it, you'll be the beloved host of your block, and people will be asking, "When's the next gathering?" (Hint: They'll probably bring snacks if you ask nicely.)

Try Something Outrageously New: Who Says You Can't?

Ever been curious about salsa dancing, stand-up comedy, or participating in a flash mob? Community activities offer the perfect chance to step out of your comfort zone. Sure, you might feel a little silly at first, but that's half the fun. Laugh at yourself, and you'll find that others will laugh 'with' you—not at you.

Embracing the unexpected can lead to some of the most memorable experiences. You might discover a hidden talent (or at least a hilarious story to share). Either way, it's a win.

Celebrate the Joy of Connection: Every Interaction Matters

Every hello at a community garden, every laugh shared at a trivia night, and every story exchanged at a local event weaves a tapestry of belonging. These moments remind us that life is richer when shared. It's not about the number of activities you do, it's about the quality of the connections you make along the way.

The magic of community isn't in the grand gestures; it's in the small, everyday moments of kindness and connection. It's the friendly wave from your neighbour, the group cheer at a fundraiser, or the collective groan when someone steals the last good bingo card.

Final Thoughts on Community Engagement: Go Forth and Mingle

Engaging with community activities is like jumping into a pool of purpose, joy, and hilarity. Sure, you might feel a bit awkward at first, but that's part of the charm. The key is to say yes—to invitations, to opportunities, to new experiences.

So, put on your "why not?" hat, step out the door, and let the community spirit sweep you off your feet. Laugh at your missteps, savor the connections, and relish the simple, profound joy of being part of something bigger than yourself. After all, life's too short to sit on the sidelines when there's so much fun to be had.

How Positive Psychology And Resilience Can Keep You Youthful

Let's start with the ultimate secret to staying young: it's not about hunting down the elusive fountain of youth, bathing in expensive serums, or stockpiling kale like it's currency for the apocalypse. Nope, the key lies in resilience—a magical, invisible force that acts like emotional bubble wrap. Resilience keeps you intact, no matter how many curveballs life hurls your way, and pairs perfectly with positive psychology, the art of focusing on the brighter side of life. Together, they're like Batman and Robin for your well-being, fighting off the villains of stress, negativity, and, dare I say, grumpiness.

Resilience: Your Emotional Bubble Wrap

Think of resilience as your personal bounce-back mechanism. It's what helps you recover from life's bumps, bruises, and downright sucker punches. Forgot where you parked the car? Resilience keeps you from spiralling into existential despair. Tripped on the sidewalk in front of a crowd? Resilience lets you laugh it off with an "I meant to do that" grin. It's like your emotional trampoline, ensuring you rebound no matter how hard the fall.

And here's the thing: resilience isn't some genetic lottery prize. It's a skill you can build, brick by brick. Studies show that resilient people are better equipped to handle stress, adapt to change, and maintain their mental sharpness (41). Resilience is the superpower that keeps you mentally spry while the rest of the world marvels at your youthful vibe.

Positive Psychology: The Glass Half-Full Perspective

Now, let's talk about positive psychology, which is essentially the VIP lounge of mental health. Instead of focusing on what's wrong, it zooms in on what's right. Positive psychology is like that friend who always finds the silver lining, even when the clouds are particularly stubborn.

This branch of psychology is less about fixing what's broken and more about nurturing joy, purpose, gratitude, and optimism. And no, it's not about faking happiness or plastering on a smile when you're feeling low. It's about genuinely cultivating the kind of mindset that makes life more enjoyable—and, as a bonus, keeps you youthful.

The Science of Staying Young (No Botox Required)

Here's the science-y bit: embracing positivity and resilience has tangible effects on your body and brain. People with a positive outlook tend to have:

Lower stress levels: Chronic stress ages us faster than a year's worth of sleepless nights.

Healthier hearts: Optimism has been linked to lower blood pressure and a reduced risk of cardiovascular disease.

Sharper minds: Resilience helps ward off cognitive decline, keeping your brain nimble.

Stronger immunity: Positivity and resilience boost your body's defences, making you less susceptible to colds, flus, and other nasties.

In short, resilience and positivity might not erase wrinkles, but they'll keep you feeling like a spring chicken long after your calendar says otherwise.

Building Resilience: The DIY Approach

If resilience were a gym, here's what your workout plan would look like:

Flex Your Gratitude Muscle: Start by jotting down three things you're thankful for every day. Even on the worst days, there's always something—like your morning coffee or the fact that you didn't trip 'twice' in public.

Shift Your Focus: Instead of dwelling on the problem, zero in on possible solutions. Lost your keys? Celebrate the extra steps you're getting while searching for them. (Fitness win!).

Learn to Laugh at Yourself: Life is way too short to take too seriously. Laugh at your mistakes, your quirks, and that time you confidently wore mismatched socks to a meeting.

Find Your Inner Zen: Mindfulness and meditation are fantastic for building resilience. Even five minutes of deep breathing can work wonders for calming your inner storm.

Connect with Others: Surround yourself with people who lift you up. A good belly laugh with friends is better than any anti-aging cream.

Positive Thinking: Your Mental Spa Day

If resilience is your emotional gym, positive thinking is like booking a day at the spa for your brain. Here's how to pamper your psyche:

Practice Kindness: A small act of kindness—whether it's holding the door for someone or complimenting a stranger's hat—can brighten your day and theirs.

Savor the Moment: Whether it's sipping your tea, watching the sunset, or just enjoying the silence, take time to relish life's little joys.

Embrace Your Inner Child: Play is not just for kids. Dance in your living room, build a sandcastle, or color outside the lines. Who cares? Life's more fun that way.

Reframe Your Thoughts: Instead of seeing challenges as roadblocks, view them as opportunities to grow. Your inner resilience coach will thank you.

The Fountain of Youth Is in Your Mindset

Here's the beauty of positive psychology and resilience: they work together to keep you vibrant, adaptable, and downright delightful. Resilience helps you weather life's storms, while positivity ensures you dance in the rain. And the best part? These tools don't come with a price tag or a pesky side effects list.

So, forget chasing eternal youth in a bottle. Instead, invest in a mindset that celebrates life's ups and downs with a twinkle in your eye and a spring in your step. After all, a youthful spirit trumps a wrinkle-free forehead any day.

Practical Takeaways for a Youthful Mindset

To sum it up:

- Laugh often, even at your own expense.

- Embrace challenges—they're character-building!

- Keep a gratitude journal, even if it's filled with silly little wins.

- Surround yourself with positive, resilient people. Energy is contagious!

Remember, the best anti-aging secret isn't found on a shelf—it's in your head and your heart.

In the end, staying youthful isn't about defying age but redefining it. With resilience and positive psychology as your secret weapons, you'll be the person everyone marvels at, wondering how you manage to stay so vibrant, light-hearted, and, well, young. Just don't forget to share your secret— or keep them guessing. Either way, you've got this.

Techniques For Resilience: Gratitude, Optimism, And Purpose

If resilience and positivity are the secret sauce to staying youthful, let's break down the recipe in glorious, technicolor detail. Like any great dish, it requires the right ingredients, and in this case, it's three life-changing techniques: gratitude, optimism, and purpose. This trifecta isn't just about surviving life's twists and turns—it's about thriving, laughing at the plot twists, and finding joy in the chaos. So, grab your apron (metaphorically speaking), and let's cook up some resilience with a hearty helping of humour.

Gratitude: A Prescription for Happiness (Side Effects May Include Smiles)

Gratitude, often touted as a shortcut to happiness, is more like finding the Wi-Fi password at a friend's house, it's life-changing once you have it. But gratitude isn't reserved for grand moments or extravagant gestures. No need to wait for a lottery win or a surprise vacation. The real magic lies in appreciating the everyday wonders: the perfect avocado, the sound of rain on a lazy afternoon, or the sweet relief of realizing you didn't forget your phone charger.

Research shows gratitude is a game-changer. It rewires your brain, lowers stress, and even improves sleep. Plus, it's contagious. Ever notice how saying "thank you" to someone often brightens their day? That's the gratitude ripple effect at work. It's like tossing kindness pebbles into the pond of life.

Gratitude in Action

The Three Things Rule: Every night before bed, jot down three things you're grateful for. They can be as small as "found the last slice of pizza" or as grand as "my team finally won." Over time, this habit shifts your focus toward the good stuff.

Gratitude Jar: Keep a jar where you drop notes of thanks for the little moments that make you smile. Revisit them when life feels heavy, it's like a greatest hits album of happiness.

Say It Out Loud: Expressing gratitude directly to someone multiplies its impact. Who doesn't like hearing, "You're awesome, and here's why"?

Remember, gratitude isn't just a fleeting feeling; it's practice. And like yoga, it's okay if you're wobbly at first—you'll get better the more you do it.

Optimism: The Power of Thinking "Why Not?" (And Sometimes "What If?")

Optimism isn't about pretending the glass is half full when it's clearly leaking. It's about acknowledging the drip while also thinking, "At least I've got a glass!" Being optimistic doesn't mean ignoring life's challenges; it's about approaching them with the mindset that there's always a solution—or at least a funny story to tell later.

Optimism has serious perks. Studies show it can boost your immune system, lower your risk of chronic diseases, and even extend your life (42, 43). Optimists aren't just people who see silver linings, they're the ones weaving them into clouds.

Optimism Hacks

Reframe the Narrative: Instead of "I can't believe I messed up," try "What a great way to learn what 'not' to do next time!"

Celebrate Small Wins: Whether it's nailing a tricky recipe or surviving a meeting without yawning, small victories deserve recognition.

Surround Yourself with Positivity: Spend time with people who lift you up, not those who drag you into the vortex of doom-scrolling. Optimism loves company.

Optimism doesn't mean life won't throw curveballs; it just means you're more likely to catch them—or at least laugh when they hit you. It's resilience's cheeky sibling, always ready to whisper, "You've got this."

Purpose: The North Star That Keeps Us Moving Forward

Ah, purpose. It's the thing that gets us out of bed in the morning—even if it's just to water that finicky houseplant or catch the sunrise. Purpose doesn't have to be monumental. You don't need to save the whales (though they'd appreciate it). Purpose is deeply personal and beautifully simple. It's about finding what makes you tick, what fills your cup, and what sparks that inner glow.

Why Purpose Matters

Living with purpose adds structure and meaning to our days. It's like a lighthouse in the fog, guiding us when life gets murky. Research confirms that people with a strong sense of purpose enjoy better health, longer lives, and more fulfilling relationships.

How to Cultivate Purpose

Follow Your Curiosity: Passion can feel like a big ask, but curiosity? That's a low stake invite to explore. Try new hobbies, volunteer for causes, or dive into topics that intrigue you.

Connect with Others: Purpose often lives in relationships. Whether it's mentoring, supporting a friend, or being the go-to dog walker in the neighborhood, connecting with others fuels a sense of significance.

Set Small Goals: Big dreams are great, but small, achievable goals give us that satisfying sense of progress. Think "write a poem," not "publish a novel."

Purpose isn't about having all the answers—it's about asking the right questions and being open to where they lead.

The Resilience Trifecta in Action: Building Your Mental Fortress

Gratitude, optimism, and purpose don't operate in isolation. Together, they form a resilience superpower that helps you tackle whatever life throws your way. Picture this:

- Gratitude grounds you. It's the foundation that reminds you there's always something good, even on the messiest days.

- Optimism lifts you. It's the boost that helps you see the potential in every challenge.

- Purpose drives you. It's the compass that keeps you moving forward, even when the path isn't clear.

When combined, they create a mental fortress—a cozy, indestructible sanctuary where you can weather any storm. And like any good fortress, it's not just about defense; it's about thriving, growing, and finding joy in the journey.

The Humour Bonus: Laughing Through It All

Let's not forget the cherry on top of the resilience sundae: humour. Finding the funny side of life is an underrated resilience booster. Laughter lightens the load and connects us with others. So, whether it's a dad joke that lands (or doesn't) or a meme that makes you snort coffee, humour is a resilience technique in its own right.

In the end, resilience isn't about being unshakable; it's about bouncing back, laughing through the wobble, and finding meaning in the journey. With gratitude, optimism, and purpose in your toolkit, you're not just surviving, you're thriving. Life may not always go according to plan, but that's okay. You've got a mental fortress, a sense of humour, and a whole lot of heart to see you through.

Mental Strength For Physical Health Over Time

Resilience, optimism, and purpose don't just keep our minds in top shape, they double as the secret sauce that helps our bodies thrive, too. Think of mental strength as the unsung hero of health, quietly working in the background to keep everything running smoothly. Unlike trendy superfoods or complicated workout routines, this magical synergy between the mind and body doesn't require a subscription, a mat, or a blender. Instead, it relies on small, consistent choices that cultivate a resilient mindset.

When you're mentally strong, you're more likely to make decisions that benefit your physical health, like choosing grilled veggies over fries (at least some of the time) or swapping a Netflix binge for a brisk walk. It's all interconnected: a clear and positive mind fuels healthy actions, which in turn keep our bodies humming happily. And yes, the 'mind-body connection' is a real thing, not just something wellness influencers toss around on Instagram.

Resilience: The Body's Quiet Cheerleader

Let's start with the star player: resilience. This isn't about pretending everything's peachy when it's not—it's about bouncing back when life throws you a curveball. Resilience helps us recover from setbacks, whether it's a bad day at work or the discovery that you've been drinking decaf by mistake.

But here's the kicker: resilience doesn't just help us emotionally; it also shields our bodies from the damaging effects of stress. Chronic stress is a sneaky villain that wreaks havoc on our hearts, disrupts sleep, and even messes with our digestion (no wonder that burrito didn't sit right!). But a resilient mindset serves as a buffer, acting like an emotional raincoat in life's downpours.

Take your cardiovascular system, for example. When you're calm and mentally strong, your heart gets a break from the constant drumbeat of stress hormones like cortisol. This keeps your blood pressure in check and reduces your risk of heart disease. In short, resilience helps your heart stay happy—both figuratively and literally.

The Power of Positivity: A Gym Membership for Your Immune System

Optimism might not cure the common cold, but it sure helps you dodge it more often. Science backs this up: people who maintain a positive outlook tend to have stronger immune systems. It's as though your body hears your positive thoughts and goes, "Alright, let's kick this into high gear!"

Think of it this way: when your mindset tells your body that everything's under control, your immune system can focus on fighting off actual threats rather than playing defense against stress- induced inflammation. Resilience acts like a coach, delivering pep talks to your immune cells, ensuring they're alert, efficient, and ready to tackle whatever comes their way.

Stress: The Aging Accelerator

Ever heard the phrase "What doesn't kill you makes you stronger"? Well, that's only partly true. Chronic stress, if left unchecked, won't kill you overnight, but it can certainly speed up the aging process. Wrinkles? Hair loss? Aches in places you didn't know existed. Blame stress for much of it.

But when you cultivate mental strength through mindfulness, gratitude, or even a daily giggle (yes, laughter is medicine!), you're giving stress the boot. Practicing gratitude, for example, can lower your blood pressure, improve sleep, and even reduce inflammation. It's like a spa day for your nervous system—minus the cucumber slices on your eyes.

Purpose: The Ultimate GPS for Life

Finding purpose is like installing a navigation system in the unpredictable journey of life. Whether it's a hobby you love, a cause you care about, or simply being there for your family, having a reason to get out of bed every morning makes a huge difference.

Purpose-driven people are more likely to stay active, socially connected, and mentally sharp, which translates to better physical health over time. And the benefits aren't just anecdotal: studies show that those with a strong sense of purpose have lower rates of heart disease and dementia (44). It's like having a life coach whispering, "Keep going—you've got this!"

Resilience Is the Glue That Holds It All Together

Building resilience isn't rocket science, but it does take a bit of effort. It's the little things that add up: deep breaths during a chaotic morning, laughing at yourself when you trip over your own feet, and choosing to see setbacks as opportunities rather than disasters.

Even better? Mental strength is contagious. Surround yourself with people who lift you up, and you'll notice your resilience growing stronger, too. Share a laugh, swap stories, or simply spend time with those who remind you to take life a little less seriously.

How Mental Strength Spurs Healthy Habits

Ever notice how a good mood makes it easier to make good choices? When you're mentally strong, you're less likely to procrastinate on things like exercise or healthy eating. That's because resilience fosters discipline. For example, instead of saying, "I'll start tomorrow," a resilient mindset encourages action now. "Sure, a jog sounds awful at first," resilience whispers, "but remember how great you felt last time?" This mental nudge is often all we need to stick to routines that benefit our bodies.

Mental Strength and Longevity: The Gift That Keeps on Giving

Here's the cherry on top: mental strength can help you live longer. Studies have found that people with positive outlooks tend to outlive their gloomier counterparts (45). Why? Because mental resilience encourages healthy living, mitigates stress, and strengthens relationships—all of which contribute to longevity.

Tips for Boosting Mental Strength (and Your Health!)

Practice Gratitude: Start or end your day by listing three things you're grateful for. Gratitude rewires your brain to focus on the positives, which reduces stress and boosts immunity.

Stay Active: Physical activity isn't just for your muscles; it's also a powerful tool for mental clarity. A simple walk in the park can clear your head and release endorphins.

Laugh Often: Humour is a free, effective stressbuster. Watch a comedy, share a joke, or laugh at your own clumsiness.

Build a Support Network: Lean on friends and family when times get tough. Connection is a powerful antidote to stress and loneliness.

Find a Passion: Whether it's painting, gardening, or perfecting your sourdough recipe, hobbies give your mind purpose and joy.

The Feel-Good Loop: Why Mental Strength and Physical Health Are Best Friends

The relationship between mental strength and physical health isn't one-sided, it's a loop. Mental resilience inspires healthy behaviors, which improve physical well-being, which then reinforces a positive mindset. It's the ultimate win-win.

So, next time you're tempted to dismiss mental resilience as fluff, remember this: your mind and body are in cahoots, and they're working together to keep you at your best. Cultivate mental strength like you would a garden—with care, patience, and a healthy dose of humour. Your body (and future self) will thank you for it.

Setting Realistic, Long-Term Goals For Healthy Aging

When it comes to healthy aging, having a plan is like prepping for a marathon—one where the finish line is a vibrant, fulfilling life, not just a participation medal for existing. Sure, you could wing it and hope for the best, but that's a risky strategy. Instead, think of long-term goals as your personalized GPS, guiding you through the twists, turns, and inevitable detours of aging. And here's the good news: goal setting doesn't have to be a slog. It can be fun, empowering, and, yes, sprinkled with a bit of humour to keep things light.

Why Goals Matter

Imagine setting out on a road trip with no destination in mind. Exciting? Maybe. Efficient? Definitely not. Without goals, you might find yourself parked in "Achy-Joint Junction" or "Sluggish- Ville" instead of cruising through "Wellness City" or "Active Aging Avenue." Goals give us a sense of direction, a purpose, and a reason to lace up those sneakers or say no to that third cookie.

But here's the kicker: the best goals aren't generic; they're deeply personal. Forget what your neighbour, cousin, or favorite Instagram influencer is doing. This is about 'you'. Your goals should reflect your dreams for the future—whether that's hiking the Appalachian Trail, chasing grandkids around the backyard, or just dancing through life without gasping for air.

The Art of Being Realistic

Let's get one thing straight: lofty goals are great for motivational speeches, but for healthy aging, practicality is king. Setting your sights on "running a marathon at 90" when you've never jogged more than three steps to catch a bus is a recipe for frustration. Instead, think smaller, more actionable steps. For instance, a long-term goal like "I want to stay active and mobile" can be broken down into bite-sized chunks:

Month 1-3: Walk 15 minutes daily.

Month 4-6: Add light strength training twice a week.

By Year-End: Work up to a daily 30-minute walk.

Not only does this approach feel more manageable, but it also gives you regular victories to celebrate—because who doesn't love a good victory dance (even if it's just a shimmy)?

Making Goals Fun

Healthy aging goals don't have to feel like homework. They can, and should, be enjoyable! If you're dreading the process, it's time to rethink the goal.

- Want to improve balance? Swap the boring exercises for a salsa class.

- Hoping to eat healthier? Turn your kitchen into a test lab for exotic recipes (who knew quinoa could be fun?).

- Trying to stay mentally sharp? Join a trivia league or start writing that memoir you've been putting off.

When your goals align with activities you genuinely enjoy, sticking to them feels less like a chore and more like a treat.

Flexibility: The Secret Ingredient

Here's a reality check: life happens. Today you're hitting 10,000 steps, but next year, 5,000 might be more realistic. The trick is to adapt without guilt. Remember, healthy aging is a marathon, not a sprint (and definitely not a race against anyone else). Adjusting your goals doesn't mean you're failing; it means you're smart enough to listen to your body. Got a bad knee? Swap running for swimming. Feeling stressed? Skip the high intensity workout for a calming yoga session. Goals should evolve as you do—like a fine wine aging alongside you.

A Framework for Goal Setting

If you're ready to dive in but don't know where to start, try this simple framework:

Get Specific: A vague goal like "I want to stay healthy" is hard to track. Instead, aim for something concrete: "I will eat two servings of vegetables at every meal" or "I will practice mindfulness for 10 minutes daily."

Make It Measurable: How will you know you've succeeded? Build in metrics: "I will walk 150 minutes a week" or "I will do strength training twice a week."

Keep It Attainable: Sure, we'd all love to bench press our body weight, but is it realistic? Start small and build from there.

Stay Relevant: Your goals should align with what truly matters to you. Want to travel more? Focus on building stamina. Love gardening? Prioritize joint health.

Set Timelines: Deadlines keep us motivated. "By next spring, I'll be able to walk five miles without stopping" is a goal you can work toward.

Examples of Long-Term Goals

To get your creative juices flowing, here are some sample long-term goals for healthy aging:

- Physical: "I want to improve my strength so I can carry my groceries without help."

- Mental: "I'll read 12 books this year to keep my mind sharp."

- Social: "I'll host a monthly game night to stay connected with friends."

- Nutritional: "I'll cut down on processed foods and cook three meals a week from scratch."

Each goal is realistic, personal, and—most importantly—achievable with a little effort.

Tracking Progress

There's nothing like a good progress tracker to keep you motivated. Whether it's a journal, an app, or a simple checklist, monitoring your achievements feels incredibly rewarding. Plus, it's a great excuse to celebrate small wins along the way (and who doesn't love a reason to treat themselves?). For example:

- Kept up with daily stretches for a month? Treat yourself to a new yoga mat.

- Hit your walking goal? Reward yourself with comfy sneakers. Celebrations don't have to be big; they just have to remind you how far you've come.

Accountability: The Power of Partnerships

Let's face it—sticking to goals is easier when someone's cheering you on. Whether it's a workout buddy, a family member, or a community group, having a support system makes all the difference.

Better yet, turn accountability into a bonding experience. Challenge a friend to a "step-off," where you both aim for a certain number of steps per week. Or join a group class where your absence will be noticed. Accountability doesn't just keep you on track; it makes the journey more enjoyable.

Looking Ahead

Healthy aging isn't about perfection; it's about progress. By setting realistic, long-term goals, you're giving yourself the gift of a purposeful, fulfilling future. And while the path might have bumps, detours, and the occasional U-turn, the destination—your best, healthiest self—is worth every step.

So, grab a notebook, jot down some goals, and start mapping your journey to "Wellness City." Remember, aging is inevitable, but how you age is up to you. Make it fun, make it meaningful, and most importantly, make it 'yours'.

Turning Healthy Aging Into An Epic Adventure

Healthy aging is not a "set it and forget it" kind of gig. It's more like baking bread, you knead it (pun intended), check on it, adjust the heat if necessary, and then celebrate when it rises. Tracking your progress, celebrating even the tiniest victories, and knowing when to pivot are essential ingredients in the recipe for success. And let's be real: this process can (and should!) be just as delightful as the goals themselves.

Progress: The Joy of Watching Yourself Grow

Tracking progress can feel like being your own personal cheerleader. It's a way of documenting your wins—big and small—while also keeping you honest about what's working and what might need tweaking. Think of it as a treasure map where the X marks your goals, and the dotted line is your journey.

But let's ditch the notion that tracking has to be some intricate system involving color-coded spreadsheets, pie charts, and graphs worthy of a NASA presentation. Nope. Simplicity is the secret sauce. A journal with bullet points will do the trick—like "Did 5 squats today and didn't fall over!" Or you're an app aficionado who likes seeing all those steps, sleep hours, or water-intake stats adding up. Prefer a more analog approach? Try the fridge calendar with colorful stickers—because let's face it, who doesn't love stickers?

The real magic lies in consistency. Make tracking a fun ritual, like your morning coffee or your evening wind-down. When you see those small accomplishments pile up, it's like binge-watching a show where you're the star.

Celebrating Small Wins: The Party Starts Now

Here's a fact: healthy aging is not a chore. It's a party, and every milestone is a reason to celebrate. If you made it around the block without wheezing, give yourself a mental high-five. Cooked a healthy dinner instead of ordering greasy takeout? That's worthy of a round of applause.

Celebrations don't have to involve confetti cannons (although, wouldn't that be fun?). They can be as simple as treating yourself to a relaxing bath, indulging in that fancy herbal tea you've been eyeing, or spending 20 guilt-free minutes with your favorite guilty-pleasure TV show. Rewards keep the journey exciting, but they also reinforce positive behavior—like training a golden retriever, except you're the adorable pup.

If you're feeling bold, involve others in your celebrations. Share your wins with a friend, a family member, or even your social media tribe. A quick "Guess who crushed their daily steps goal today? This person!" post can bring in a flurry of supportive likes, comments, and virtual fist bumps.

Adjusting: When Life Throws Curveballs

Here's the thing about life—it doesn't always cooperate with your plans. You wake up with a twinge in your back, or your calendar gets hijacked by unexpected responsibilities. These moments can feel like setbacks, but in the grand adventure of healthy aging, they're actually plot twists.

Adjusting your goals isn't admitting defeat; it's being smart. If you've been aiming for 10,000 steps a day but your knees are protesting, scaling back to 6,000 is not failure—it's wisdom. Remember, healthy aging is not a sprint; it's the scenic route where you occasionally pull over to admire the view. The key to adjusting is keeping a growth mindset. Every challenge is a chance to learn more about yourself, your limits, your resilience, and your ability to adapt. You discover that yoga is a better fit for your current energy level than that high-intensity spin class. Or you realize that a short walk is just as satisfying as a long one on days when you're pressed for time.

Adjusting is also about listening to your body. You wouldn't ignore your car's "check engine" light (at least, not for long), so why ignore your body's signals? If something feels off, it's okay to pause, reassess, and reset. The goal isn't perfection; it's progress over time.

Making It a Habit: Routine Meets Spontaneity

One of the biggest challenges in tracking, celebrating, and adjusting is sticking with it. This is where routines come to the rescue. Build healthy aging habits into your daily life so that they become as automatic as brushing your teeth.

For example, turn your tracking into a bedtime ritual: "Today I stretched for 15 minutes and resisted the cookies at lunch. Go me!" Or make celebrations part of your week: "Friday is reward day, and I'm treating myself to a walk by the lake with a coffee afterward." But here's the twist —don't let routine turn into monotony. Sprinkle in some spontaneity to keep things lively. Try a new healthy recipe, explore a different walking route, or swap your usual yoga session for a dance class. Surprises keep the journey exciting and ensure you're always looking forward to what's next.

The Power of Reflection: Looking Back to Move Forward

Every so often, take a moment to reflect on how far you've come. You started with the goal of walking 15 minutes a day, and now you're comfortably doing 45. You've gone from "barely surviving" a workout to actually looking forward to it. Reflection isn't just about patting yourself on the back, it's also about recharging your motivation for the road ahead. Reflection can also help you spot trends. You notice that your energy dips in the afternoon, so you switch your workouts to the morning. Or you realize that your progress stalls when you don't get enough sleep, prompting you to prioritize rest. These insights are like breadcrumbs guiding you toward even better strategies.

Tracking and Celebrating: A Recipe for Longevity

Healthy aging is about enjoying the ride, not just the destination. When you track your progress, you're acknowledging every step forward. When you celebrate your wins, you're injecting joy into the process. And when you adjust as needed, you're proving to yourself that flexibility is your secret weapon.

So, whether you're smashing your fitness goals or taking baby steps toward them, remember to savor every moment. After all, the best adventures aren't the ones where everything goes perfectly—they're the ones where you adapt, grow, and come out smiling on the other side. And who knows? You might even inspire someone else to start their own healthy aging journey. Now that's worth celebrating.

Goal-Setting Exercises And Motivational Tips

With the basics of goal setting down pat, it's time to roll up our sleeves (or hiking pants) and dive into practical goal-setting exercises and motivational tips. Healthy aging isn't about grim determination, it's about mixing a little strategy with a lot of joy. Think of it as a choose-your-own- adventure story, where every choice you make adds more vibrancy to the years ahead. So, grab a notebook (or your favorite app) and let's get started with tools to help you age like the legend you are.

Exercise 1: The "One Thing" Exercise – Small Wins, Big Gains

Let's keep it simple to start: What's one thing you can do today that your future self will thank you for? Seriously, just one. It could be drinking a glass of water first thing in the morning instead of coffee, standing up to stretch after an hour of sitting, or choosing the stairs instead of the elevator. These tiny actions are like pennies in the piggy bank of aging well—they add up over time.

Pro tip: Treat your "one thing" as a non-negotiable date with yourself. Put it on your calendar, give it a name like "Future-You Fuel," and celebrate it with a little fist pump when you've done it. One small thing a day? That's 365 healthy choices a year. That's practically a master's degree in aging well!

Exercise 2: The "Why" Drill-Down – Get to the Heart of It

A goal without a purpose is like a smoothie without the fruit—bland and unmotivating. So, let's play detective and uncover your real motivation. Start with your goal. Say it's "I want to exercise more." Ask yourself why. You say, "To feel stronger." Then ask why again. "Because I want to keep playing with my grandkids." Keep digging until you hit your "aha" moment—your true driving force. Example:

Goal: "I want to eat more vegetables."

Why? "To stay healthy."

Why? "So, I can avoid chronic illness."

Why? "Because I want to travel the world when I retire."

Boom. Now you're not just munching on kale; you're fuelling adventures in Tuscany and beyond.

Exercise 3: The Buddy System – Because Everything's Better with a Friend

Aging well is a team sport. Enlist a buddy—someone who shares your enthusiasm (or at least pretends to). Whether it's a weekly walk, swapping recipes, or a Zoom yoga session, having someone to share your journey with makes it infinitely more fun.

No local buddy? No problem! Online communities are a treasure trove of support. Join groups with people pursuing similar goals. Share your wins, laugh about your fails, and soak up the collective energy of people rooting for each other.

Bonus tip: Make it competitive. "Who hit 10,000 steps first this week?" or "Who tried the weirdest new vegetable?" (Pro tip: Romanesco looks like alien broccoli and tastes divine!)

Motivational Tip 1: Visualize Your Future Self – The Inner Motivational Speaker

Close your eyes and picture Future You. What do they look like? (Hopefully, they're not glaring back at you for skipping the stretching session again.) Instead, imagine a vibrant, active version of yourself, hiking through the mountains, dancing at a family wedding, or simply bending over to tie your shoes without grunting. Future You is the person you're working for today. Keep that image clear in your mind. On tough days, ask yourself, "What would Future Me want me to do right now?" (Spoiler: It's probably not watching three hours of cat videos, unless you're doing yoga stretches at the same time.)

Motivational Tip 2: Mantras and Affirmations – Words to Live By

Mantras are like little pep talks you carry in your pocket. They're easy to whip out when motivation dips. Create a mantra that feels personal and inspiring. Here are a few to get you started:

- "Strong today, stronger tomorrow."

- "Every step is progress."

- "Healthy aging is a choice, and I choose it daily."

Write your mantra on sticky notes, set it as your phone wallpaper, or shout it into the void while jogging. Repetition makes it stick—and keeps you focused on the big picture.

Exercise 4: The "Treasure Map" Vision Board – Plot Your Aging Adventure

Why let the 20-somethings have all the vision-board fun? Create a "treasure map" for your healthy aging journey. Clip pictures, jot down words, and stick-up photos that represent your goals. Whether it's an image of a serene yoga pose, a passport for your dream destinations, or a vegetable garden bursting with produce, this is your visual reminder of where you're headed. Hang it somewhere you'll see every day. It's harder to skip that salad when your treasure map whispers, "Tuscany isn't ready for you yet."

Motivational Tip 3: Make Friends with Failure – It's Just Feedback

Here's the deal: You're going to slip up. You skip a workout or devour a pint of ice cream during a Netflix binge. The key is not to see these moments as failures but as feedback. What went wrong? Were you too tired? Stressed? Did you need more support? Reflect, adjust, and move forward. Healthy aging isn't about perfection; it's about persistence. Besides, life's more interesting with a few plot twists, right?

Exercise 5: The Goal Jar – A Lucky Dip for Your Future

Take a jar and fill it with mini goals on slips of paper. Each week, pull one out and focus on it. Examples might include "Try one new vegetable," "Walk an extra 1,000 steps," or "Do 10 minutes of mindfulness." This gamifies goal setting, turning healthy aging into a fun, weekly challenge. Plus, who doesn't love a good surprise?

Motivational Tip 4: Celebrate the Wins – Big or Small

Milestones are meant to be celebrated. Hit your goal of drinking 8 glasses of water a day? Treat yourself to a fancy reusable water bottle. Stuck to your weekly walks for a month? Grab a new pair of sneakers. Celebration keeps you motivated and reminds you that you're making progress.

Pro Tip: Keep a journal of your victories. On low-motivation days, flip back through and remind yourself how far you've come. Spoiler: You're awesome.

Exercise 6: Monthly Reflect and Reset – Stay Agile

Healthy aging is a living process, so your goals should evolve with you. Every month, take 10 minutes to review your progress. What's working? What isn't? What needs a tweak? This keeps your goals fresh and relevant while allowing you to celebrate your progress—or pivot if necessary.

Final Thought: A Journey Worth Taking

Healthy aging isn't about following a strict script—it's an improvisational dance through life's later years. These exercises and tips are tools to help you stay focused, have fun, and keep moving forward. Remember, every choice is a step in the right direction, and every step brings you closer to living your best life.

So go ahead: set those goals, laugh at the inevitable hiccups, and keep visualizing that vibrant, thriving version of yourself. After all, healthy aging isn't just about adding years to your life; it's about adding life to your years.

CHAPTER 15: BLUEPRINT FOR A FRAILTY-FREE FUTURE

The Key Takeaways

Congratulations, fearless reader! You've not only survived but thrived on this odyssey toward a healthier, frailty-free future. Along the way, we've tackled everything from embracing positivity to mastering balance—and yes, even how to laugh in the face of aging (wrinkles included). Now it's time for a stroll down memory lane as we unpack the golden nuggets from each chapter. Think of this as your ultimate cheat sheet to becoming the lively, resilient rock star of your golden years. Ready? Let's dive in!

Embracing Aging With Positivity

Aging is less about counting candles on your cake and more about the glow in your heart. Science says a positive mindset isn't just for the glass-half-full crowd, it's a secret weapon for well-being. Wrinkles? Nah, those are just laugh lines proving you've lived (and laughed) well. So, slap on that metaphorical (or literal) sunscreen, smile wide, and let your inner optimist shine brighter than your neighbour's lawn ornaments.

The Power Of Movement

Exercise isn't reserved for spandex-wearing gym-goers. Whether it's dancing at a wedding or weeding the garden, movement is your BFF. Keep your body in motion, and it'll reward you with more energy, better mobility, and the ability to reach for the cookie jar without pulling a muscle. Pro tip: Pick activities you genuinely love. Nothing beats burning calories while belly-laughing through Zumba class.

Building Bone Strength

Bones aren't just structural; they're the unsung heroes of your "let's stay upright" mission. Calcium and vitamin D are the power couple of bone health, and weight-bearing exercises (think: walking, dancing) are their sidekicks. Strong bones don't just help you stand tall; they keep you resilient, like a skyscraper in a windstorm.

Brain Health And Cognitive Vitality

Your brain is the command center of your fabulous self, so keep it sharp! Think puzzles, learning new hobbies, or debating whether pineapple belongs on pizza (it does!). Social activities are like Zumba for your neurons, and curiosity keeps your gray matter firing on all cylinders. Stay mentally spry and you'll be the life of every trivia night.

Building Strength And Flexibility

We're not saying you need Hulk-level muscles, but a little strength goes a long way. Strong muscles and supple joints keep you independent and out of the "help, I've fallen, and I can't get up" infomercial. Squats, yoga, or a gentle stretch in the morning—whatever floats your boat—are all investments in your body's stock market of freedom.

Nourishing Your Body For Longevity

Your body is a temple, not a trash can for leftover pizza crusts (okay, occasionally). Fuel it with lean proteins, colorful veggies, and a rainbow of fruits. Not only will your energy soar, but your skin might just radiate enough to save on nightlights. Bonus points for staying hydrated—because water is the MVP of health, glowing skin, and fighting off cranky moods.

Sleep Smart

Sleep isn't just for laziness, it's where your body repairs, recharges, and dreams about vacation destinations. Quality shut eye makes everything better: mood, memory, and even your ability to tolerate your morning alarm. Embrace your inner slumber champion, and don't skimp on those Zs. You deserve it, dreamer extraordinaire.

Heart Health Essentials

Your heart doesn't just keep you alive; it's your dance partner for all of life's best moments. Moderate exercise—hello, brisk walks—and a dash of stress management keep your ticker in tip-top shape. Pair that with a diet low in processed foods and high in love, and you're set to waltz your way into a long, healthy life.

Managing Stress With Style

Stress happens—it's life's way of keeping things interesting. But managing it is where the magic lies. Deep breaths, a solid playlist, and a little humour go a long way. Remember, you're the calm captain of your ship, sailing through turbulent seas. And when in doubt, laughter truly is the best medicine.

Balance And Coordination

Balance isn't just for tightrope walkers. It's your safeguard against tumbles and stumbles. Simple exercises, like standing on one leg or yoga poses, make all the difference. Build your balance today, and you'll be the graceful swan of the family reunion instead of the clumsy cousin.

Social Health

Humans are social creatures, and friendships are like sunshine for the soul. Whether it's chatting with friends, joining a club, or laughing until your cheeks hurt, staying socially active keeps loneliness at bay and happiness on tap. Your laughter-filled hangouts are secret superfoods for your health.

in your future self. So, lace up those sneakers, even if they're a little dusty. Call that friend you've been meaning to catch up with. Dance like nobody's watching (and if they are, give them a good show). Each of these acts is a declaration that life, in all its messy, unpredictable glory, is worth showing up for.

The Resilient Legacy

Here's the big picture: resilience isn't just for you. It's a legacy you pass on to others. By living a resilient life, you're showing your loved ones—whether they're your kids, grandkids, or friends—that life's challenges are opportunities for growth, not reasons to give up. And remember, resilience isn't about being perfect or fearless. It's about being brave enough to try, strong enough to adapt, and wise enough to laugh when things don't go as planned.

A Toast to Resilience

So, here's to you and the resilient spirit you're building, one small act at a time. May it carry you through life's ups and downs, fill your days with laughter, and remind you that the best is yet to come. Whether you're climbing a metaphorical mountain or just trying to figure out how to use your new fitness tracker, know that resilience is your trusty sidekick, always ready to help you rise to the occasion. Because let's face it: life's too short not to thrive—and resilience is your ticket to doing just that. Cheers to a lifetime of strength, joy, and the endless adventure of living well!

CEO: Chief Executive Officer

CFS: Clinical Frailty Scale

CGA: Comprehensive Geriatric Assessment

DHL: Dalsey, Hillblom, and Lynn

DM: Diabetes mellitus

FedEx: Federal Express

FFP: Fried Frailty Phenotype

FI: Frailty Index

HIIT: High-Intensity Interval Training

IBS: Irritable Bowel Syndrome

MVP: Most Valuable Player

PTA: Parent-Teacher Association

REM: Rapid Eye Movement

REFERENCES

1. Fried LP, Tangen CM, Walston J, Newman AB, Hirsch C, Gottdiener J. Frailty in older adults: evidence for a phenotype. J Gerontol A Biol Sci Med Sci. 2001; 56.

2. Mitnitski AB, Mogilner AJ, Rockwood K. Accumulation of deficits as a proxy measure of aging. Scient World J. 2001; 1: 323-36.

3. Cesari M, Gambassi G, Abellan Van Kan G, Vellas B. The frailty phenotype and the frailty index: different instruments for different purposes. Age and Ageing. 2014;43 (1): 10-2.

4. Walston J, Hadley EC, Ferrucci L, Guralnik JM, Newman AB, Studenski SA, et al. Research agenda for frailty in older adults: toward a better understanding of physiology and etiology: summary from the American Geriatrics Society/ National Institute on Aging Research Conference on Frailty in Older Adults. J Am Geriatr Soc. 2006;54 (6): 991-1001.

5. Dent E, Kowal P, Hoogendijk EO. Frailty measurement in research and clinical practice: A review. European Journal of Internal Medicine. 2016; 31: 3-10.

6. Gale CR, Westbury L, Cooper C. Social isolation and loneliness as risk factors for the progression of frailty: the English Longitudinal Study of Ageing. Age and Ageing. 2017; 47 (3): 392-7.

7. Marcucci M, Damanti S, Germini F, Apostolo J, Bobrowicz-Campos E, Gwyther H, et al. Interventions to prevent, delay or reverse frailty in older people: a journey towards clinical guidelines. BMC Medicine. 2019; 17 (1): 193.

8. Rockwood K, Mitnitski A. Frailty in Relation to the Accumulation of Deficits. The Journals of Gerontology: Series A. 2007; 62 (7): 722-7.

9. Merchant RA, Aprahamian I, Woo J, Vellas B, Morley JE. Editorial: Resilience And Successful Aging. J Nutr Health Aging. 2022; 26 (7): 652-6.

10. Ebeling PR, Daly RM, Kerr DA, Kimlin MG. Building healthy bones throughout life: an evidence-informed strategy to prevent osteoporosis in Australia. Medical Journal of Australia. 2013; 199 (S7): S1-S46.

11. Posadzki P, Pieper D, Bajpai R, Makaruk H, Könsgen N, Neuhaus AL, et al. Exercise/physical activity and health outcomes: an overview of Cochrane systematic reviews. BMC Public Health. 2020; 20 (1): 1724.

12. Verghese J, Lipton RB, Katz MJ, Hall CB, Derby CA, Kuslansky G, et al. Leisure activities and the risk of dementia in the elderly. N Engl J Med. 2003; 348 (25): 2508-16.

13. Ye L, Bally E, Korenhof SA, Fierloos I, Alhambra Borrás T, Clough G, et al. The association between loneliness and frailty among community-dwelling older adults in five European countries: a longitudinal study. Age and Ageing. 2024; 53 (10).

14. Cardona M, Andrés P. Are social isolation and loneliness associated with cognitive decline in ageing? Frontiers in Aging Neuroscience. 2023; 15.

15. Hawkley LC, Cacioppo JT. Loneliness matters: a theoretical and empirical review of consequences and mechanisms. Ann Behav Med. 2010;40 (2): 218-27.

16. Boss L, Kang D-H, Branson S. Loneliness and cognitive function in the older adult: a systematic review. International Psychogeriatrics. 2015; 27 (4): 541-53.

17. Borges MK, Canevelli M, Cesari M, Aprahamian I. Frailty as a Predictor of Cognitive Disorders: A Systematic Review and Meta-Analysis. Frontiers in Medicine. 2019; 6.

18. Bandeen-Roche K, Seplaki CL, Huang J, Buta B, Kalyani RR, Varadhan R, et al. Frailty in Older Adults: A Nationally Representative Profile in the United States. J Gerontol A Biol Sci Med Sci. 2015; 70 (11): 1427- 34.

19. Ekram ARMS, Tonkin AM, Ryan J, Beilin L, Ernst ME, Espinoza SE, et al. The association between frailty and incident cardiovascular disease events in community-dwelling healthy older adults. Am Heart J Plus. 2023; 28.

20. Veronese N, Koyanagi A, Smith L, Musacchio C, Cammalleri L, Barbagallo M, et al. Multidimensional frailty increases cardiovascular risk in older people: An 8-year longitudinal cohort study in the Osteoarthritis Initiative. Experimental Gerontology. 2021; 147: 111265.

21. Theou O, Rockwood MR, Mitnitski A, Rockwood K. Disability and co-morbidity in relation to frailty: how much do they overlap? Arch Gerontol Geriatr. 2012; 55 (2): e1-8.

22. Ekram ARMS, Ryan J, Espinoza S, Newman AB, Murray AM, Orchard SG, et al. The association between frailty and dementia-free and physical disability-free survival in community-dwelling older adults. Gerontology. 2023.

23. Majid Z, Welch C, Davies J, Jackson T. Global frailty: The role of ethnicity, migration and socioeconomic factors. Maturitas. 2020; 139: 33-41.

24. Hoogendijk EO, Heymans MW, Deeg DJH, Huisman M. Socioeconomic Inequalities in Frailty among Older Adults: Results from a 10-Year Longitudinal Study in the Netherlands. Gerontology. 2018; 64 (2): 157-64.

25. Xu W, Tan C-C, Zou J-J, Cao X-P, Tan L. Sleep problems and risk of all-cause cognitive decline or dementia: an updated systematic review and meta-analysis. Journal of Neurology, Neurosurgery & Amp; Amp; Psychiatry. 2020; 91 (3): 236.

26. Kong J, Zhou L, Li X, Ren Q. Sleep disorders affect cognitive function in adults: an overview of systematic reviews and meta-analyses. Sleep and Biological Rhythms. 2023; 21 (2): 133-42.

27. Kramer CK, Leitao CB. Laughter as medicine: A systematic review and meta-analysis of interventional studies evaluating the impact of spontaneous laughter on cortisol levels. PLOS ONE. 2023; 18 (5): e0286260.

28. Woo J, Goggins W, Sham A, Ho SC. Social determinants of frailty. Gerontology. 2005; 51 (6): 402-8.

29. Peleg O, Peleg M. Is Resilience the Bridge Connecting Social and Family Factors to Mental

Well-Being and Life Satisfaction? Contemporary Family Therapy. 2024.

30. Boyes A 2018; Pages: https://www.psychologytoday.com/us/blog/in-practice/201802/6-benefits- uncluttered space on 17 December 2024.

31. American Psychological Association 2020; Pages: https://www.apa.org/topics/ exercise-fitness/stress on 17 December 2024.

32. Cook JD, Charest J. Sleep and Performance in Professional Athletes. Current Sleep Medicine Reports. 2023; 9 (1): 56-81.

33. Cunha LA, Costa JA, Marques EA, Brito J, Lastella M, Figueiredo P. The Impact of Sleep Interventions on Athletic Performance: A Systematic Review. Sports Medicine - Open. 2023; 9 (1): 58.

34. Lee DH, Rezende LFM, Joh H-K, Keum N, Ferrari G, Rey-Lopez JP, et al. Long-Term Leisure-Time Physical Activity Intensity and All-Cause and Cause-Specific Mortality: A Prospective Cohort of US Adults. Circulation. 2022; 146 (7): 523-34.

35. Mandsager K, Harb S, Cremer P, Phelan D, Nissen SE, Jaber W. Association of Cardiorespiratory Fitness With Long-term Mortality Among Adults Undergoing Exercise Treadmill Testing. JAMA Network Open. 2018; 1 (6): e183605-e.

36. Lang JJ, Prince SA, Merucci K, Cadenas-Sanchez C, Chaput J-P, Fraser BJ, et al. Cardiorespiratory fitness is a strong and consistent predictor of morbidity and mortality among adults: an overview of meta- analyses representing over 20.9 million observations from 199 unique cohort studies. British Journal of Sports Medicine. 2024; 58 (10): 556.

37. Lee B-A, Oh D-J. The effects of long-term aerobic exercise on cardiac structure, stroke volume of the left ventricle, and cardiac output. J Exerc Rehabil. 2016; 12 (1): 37-41.

38. Blomstrand P, Tesan D, Nylander EM, Ramstrand N. Mind body exercise improves cognitive function more than aerobic- and resistance exercise in healthy adults aged 55 years and older – an umbrella review. European Review of Aging and Physical Activity. 2023; 20 (1): 15.

39. Vila J. Social Support and Longevity: Meta-Analysis-Based Evidence and Psychobiological Mechanisms. Front Psychol. 2021; 12: 717164.

40. Holt-Lunstad J, Smith TB, Layton JB. Social Relationships and Mortality Risk: A Meta-analytic Review. PLOS Medicine. 2010; 7 (7): e1000316.

41. Joyce S, Shand F, Tighe J, Laurent SJ, Bryant RA, Harvey SB. Road to resilience: a systematic review and meta-analysis of resilience training programmes and interventions. BMJ Open. 2018; 8(6): e017858.

42. Schiavon CC, Marchetti E, Gurgel LG, Busnello FM, Reppold CT. Optimism and Hope in Chronic Disease: A Systematic Review. Front Psychol. 2016; 7: 2022.

43. Koga HK, Trudel-Fitzgerald C, Lee LO, James P, Kroenke C, Garcia L, et al. Optimism, lifestyle, and longevity in a racially diverse cohort of women. J Am Geriatr Soc. 2022; 70 (10): 2793-804.

44. Bell G, Singham T, Saunders R, John A, Stott J. Positive psychological constructs and association with reduced risk of mild cognitive impairment and dementia in older adults: A

Embracing Mobility And Independence

Mobility equals freedom. Whether it's strengthening your legs, improving posture, or simply remembering to stand tall, keeping mobile lets you write your own story. Need a cane or assistance? That's not a setback; it's a tool to keep you rocking the independence vibe. Mobility isn't just about moving, it's about living.

Mental Resilience

Aging gracefully is as much about the mind as the body. Resilience comes from gratitude, optimism, and finding purpose. Practice kindness—to yourself and others—and you'll discover that every gray hair is a badge of wisdom earned through resilience and grace.

Goal Setting For The Long Haul

Goals are like GPS coordinates for your life. Whether it's running a 5K or mastering a new hobby, realistic, flexible goals keep you motivated. Track your progress, celebrate small wins, and remember aging well isn't a sprint, it's a joyful, leisurely marathon. And guess what? You're already winning.

Revolutionizing Frailty Care: Meds, Tech, And Policies

While healthy lifestyle encompassing physical activity, diet, and social interactions are often highlighted in discussions about aging, there are other evidence-based interventions that can make a real difference in improving frailty status and health outcomes for older adults.

Pharmacological Treatments

Medications can play a key role in managing chronic conditions that commonly affect older adults, such as hypertension, diabetes mellitus, and osteoporosis. For example, drugs like statins and blood pressure medications help reduce the risk of cardiovascular disease, while bisphosphonates strengthen bones and reduce fractures. In addition, medications like cognitive enhancers may slow the progression of dementia in some cases. Proper medication management can significantly improve quality of life and help older adults maintain independence for longer.

In the future, medications targeting frailty itself—such as agents that address muscle loss, inflammation, or hormonal imbalances—could further enhance care, offering new hope for preventing or reversing frailty's effects.

Assistive Technologies

Tools like mobility aids, hearing aids, and smart devices can dramatically improve the day-to-day lives of older adults. From simple walkers that provide stability to high-tech home monitoring systems that detect falls or manage chronic diseases remotely, assistive technologies support aging in place and prevent hospitalizations. Devices such as voice-controlled home assistants and wearable health trackers also offer greater autonomy and peace of mind, empowering older adults to take charge of their health. In the future, innovations like robotic exoskeletons to aid movement and artificial intelligence to predict and prevent health crises may revolutionize care, allowing older adults to stay active and independent longer.

Policy-Level Solutions

Governments and communities can make a big impact by creating environments that support aging well. Age-friendly policies include making public spaces more accessible, offering transportation options for those with limited mobility, and ensuring that homes and buildings are designed with safety in mind. Urban planning that prioritizes walkability, access to healthcare services, and social engagement fosters well-being and reduces isolation. Creating policies that promote affordable healthcare, social services, and community-building can significantly enhance the health and quality of life for older adults. Well-designed policies that integrate care for frailty, like funding for preventive services and home-based care, could be a game-changer in ensuring that older adults maintain their independence and dignity.

However, detailed discussions on pharmacological interventions, assistive technologies and policy-level solutions are beyond the scope of this book. Each of these interventions, when combined with a healthy lifestyle, builds a comprehensive approach to aging that supports long-term health, independence, and dignity.

Healthy aging isn't about chasing perfection. It's about creating a life where you can laugh easily, move freely, and embrace the years ahead with gusto. Each chapter in this book has been a stepping stone toward that vision. So go ahead, fearless reader, and tackle your golden years with a heart full of gratitude, a mind bursting with resilience, and a body ready for the adventures to come. Because the best is yet to be!

A Simple, Step-By-Step Action Plan You Can Start Today

Are you ready to embark on your journey toward a vibrant, frailty-free future? Don't worry, you don't need to reinvent yourself overnight or become a kale-worshipping yoga guru by tomorrow morning. This plan is as easy as it is enjoyable, designed to fit seamlessly into your life. Think of it as upgrading to the deluxe version of you, one delightful, manageable step at a time.

Set Your Vision: Dream Big, But Not Bonkers

Picture this: It's 10 years from now, and you're dancing at a family wedding, conquering a mountain trail, or finally nailing that tricky yoga pose that's been on your bucket list. Visualization is like a sneak peek into your future—and a powerful motivator to take the first step.

Take a moment to jot down your vision of a thriving, healthy self. Make it personal, vivid, and even a little cheeky. Forget about society's version of "aging gracefully" (spoiler: it often involves overpriced creams). Instead, focus on your own goals, whether it's being able to lift your groceries without breaking a sweat or mastering the art of stress-free mornings.

Get Moving Daily: It's Like a Happy Dance for Your Body

We're not talking marathon training here—unless that's your jam. Start small. Movement should feel like a gift to your body, not a punishment for that second slice of pie. If you're starting from scratch, try a gentle 10-minute walk around your block or a stretch session that doubles as an excuse to binge-watch your favorite show ("Downward Dog" during a sitcom? Genius). If you're already active, kick it up a notch—take the stairs, try a new class, or dust off those roller skates.

The secret sauce? Consistency. Aim for something you can actually look forward to, whether that's grooving to your favorite playlist or recruiting your dog as a workout buddy (bonus points if you both wear matching headbands).

Fuel with Purpose: Your Taste Buds and Body Can Be Friends

Healthy eating isn't about deprivation; it's about small, satisfying swaps. Start by adding one extra veggie to your plate. Broccoli in pasta? Yes. Spinach in smoothies? Absolutely. You'll feel like a culinary wizard without breaking a sweat.

Cutting back on sugar doesn't mean exiling dessert to the land of forgotten pleasures. Swap cookies for dark chocolate, soda for sparkling water, or chips for crunchy chickpeas. It's all about finding the middle ground between indulgence and nourishment.

Oh, and don't forget hydration! If plain water feels like a chore, jazz it up with slices of cucumber, mint, or a splash of citrus. You're not just drinking water—you're sipping on a spa day.

Connect with a Friend: Your Secret Anti-Aging Elixir

Loneliness ages you faster than a sunbathing habit in the '90s. The antidote? Connection. Call an old friend, schedule a coffee date, or join a club that intrigues you (book club? gardening? underwater basket weaving?).

Socializing isn't just fun; it's good for your brain and heart. Plus, who doesn't love a good laugh? Pro tip: Double the benefits by combining movement with connection—take a walking meeting or sign up for a group fitness class.

If meeting in person isn't an option, embrace technology. A quick video call with your favorite human can boost your mood faster than your morning coffee.

Challenge Your Brain: Because Gray Cells Need TLC Too

Your brain loves a good workout as much as your body does. Keep it sharp with puzzles, trivia, or learning a new skill. Ever tried knitting? Chess? Salsa dancing? They're not just hobbies; they're secret weapons against cognitive decline.

Carve out time daily—even if it's just five minutes—to engage your brain. And if you're feeling ambitious, consider learning a new language or mastering a musical instrument. The goal isn't perfection; it's keeping your neurons nimble.

Start a Gratitude Journal: A Dose of Happy Before Bed

Gratitude isn't just a warm, fuzzy feeling, it's a full-on wellness strategy. Grab a notebook and scribble down three things you're thankful for each evening. They can be big (family, health) or small (a really good cup of coffee, your neighbour's adorable dog).

Science backs this one: practicing gratitude improves your mood, helps you sleep better, and even boosts your immune system. Bonus? It's free. No subscriptions, no equipment, just pure positivity.

Balance and Strength Practice: Your Future Self Will Thank You

Nobody wants to be that person who trips over nothing. Balance and strength exercises are your ticket to stability and confidence, not to mention fewer bruises. Start small. Can you stand on one foot while brushing your teeth? Voilà—a multitasking marvel. Add simple strength moves like squats, lunges, or push-ups against the wall. These mini sessions add up to major gains over time.

The key is consistency. Five minutes a day is all it takes to build a foundation that'll keep you upright and independent well into your golden years.

Sleep Smarter: Snooze Like a Pro

Sleep isn't just downtime—it's your body's repair and recharge mode. Aim for 7–9 hours a night and treat bedtime like the sacred ritual it is. Set a consistent schedule, wind down with calming activities (a good book, meditation, or your favorite low-drama podcast), and keep screens out of sight. If sleep eludes you, try a warm bath, chamomile tea, or a little bedtime yoga. And remember, naps aren't just for toddlers, they're a secret weapon for recharging midday. Just keep them short (20 minutes max) to avoid messing with your nighttime sleep.

Celebrate Every Win: High-Five Yourself

Don't wait for monumental achievements to celebrate. Every step forward, no matter how small, is worth a mini celebration. Did you hit your step goal for the day? Treat yourself to a bubble bath. Tried a new recipe? Snap a pic and share it with friends.

Celebrating creates a positive feedback loop. You'll associate healthy habits with happiness and be more likely to stick with them. Plus, who doesn't love an excuse to throw an occasional dance party in the kitchen?

Keep It Fun and Flexible: Your Plan, Your Rules

Healthy aging isn't about rigid schedules or unrealistic expectations. It's about creating a life that feels good, one small step at a time. Life happens—adjust your plan as needed. If a goal isn't working, tweak it. If you miss a day (or a week), forgive yourself and start fresh.

The most important step? Enjoy the process. Whether you're lifting weights, lifting your spirits, or lifting a fork full of salad, let it bring joy. After all, the goal isn't just to live longer, it's to live better. By starting today, you're setting the stage for a future that's vibrant, active, and full of possibilities. And remember, the journey to healthy aging is best taken one smile, one stretch, and one step at a time. Let's do this!

Motivating Message on the Lifelong Benefits of Building Resilience

Picture this: You're strolling through life like the main character in a feel-good movie, soundtrack and all, when suddenly—BAM! Life throws a curveball. It's a stiff knee, a bad day, or yet another relative sending you unsolicited "miracle cure" links. Enter resilience, your unsung superhero, cape fluttering in the wind. Resilience isn't just about bouncing back, it's about bouncing forward, stronger and wiser, like the wise-cracking protagonist who grows into their role as the story unfolds.

Resilience Is Your Secret Superpower

Resilience is like a secret weapon hidden in plain sight. It's not flashy or loud, but trust me, it's potent. Building resilience is signing up for a lifelong membership to the "I've Got This" club. It's the grit that gets you through those morning stretches when your bed feels like paradise. It's determination that helps you swap fries for salad (well, most of the time). And it's the courage that allows you to laugh when life's little absurdities come knocking.

Here's the kicker: resilience isn't something you're born with. Sure, some people seem naturally Zen, but for the rest of us mere mortals, resilience is a skill—a muscle you build through small, intentional acts of self-care, self-love, and sometimes a little trial and error.

The Snowball Effect of Small Wins

Think of resilience like a snowball rolling downhill. Each little success—whether it's mastering a yoga pose, drinking enough water, or remembering where you put your keys—adds up. Over time, these tiny victories form a giant ball of confidence that makes life's challenges seem like mere speed bumps.

Tried a new recipe and managed not to set off the smoke alarm? That's resilience. Stumbled through a Zumba class but left with a smile? Resilience again. These moments might feel small, but they're the stepping stones to a life well-lived. And the best part? Resilience has a compounding effect. The more you invest in it, the more it gives back—like the world's most reliable savings account.

Laugh Through the Chaos

One of the most underrated tools in the resilience toolkit is laughter. Got caught in the rain?

Laugh about it. Tried a trendy new exercise and ended up looking like a flailing octopus? Laugh about that too. Laughter isn't just good for the soul—it's a full-body workout for your spirit, and it helps you keep perspective when life gets tricky.

By embracing humour, you're giving yourself permission to let go of perfection. Spoiler alert: nobody's perfect, not even the person who always shows up to Pilates with perfectly matching outfits. Life is messy, unpredictable, and sometimes downright silly. Resilience is about rolling with it, often while laughing at the absurdity of it all.

Building a Resilience Routine

Here's the thing about resilience: it doesn't just show up when you need it most. You've got to nurture it, like a plant you water daily (but not the kind you accidentally forget on the windowsill). Building resilience is about creating habits that reinforce your inner strength. Start small. It takes a five-minute walk each day or swapping one sugary drink for water. Celebrate these wins. Over time, these tiny changes create a ripple effect, reshaping not just your body but your mindset.

Pro tip: Don't underestimate the power of gratitude. Jotting down a few things you're grateful for each day is like doing push-ups for your soul. It trains your brain to focus on the positives, even when the world seems determined to test your patience.

The Resilience Ripple

Here's where it gets interesting: resilience doesn't just impact you. It's contagious. When you model resilience—by staying optimistic, handling challenges gracefully, or simply showing up for yourself, you inspire others to do the same. Your friends, family, and even that grumpy neighbour who never waves back can feel the ripple effect of your resilience. And let's talk about the long game. Building resilience isn't just about surviving the tough days; it's about thriving in the face of them. It's the foundation for healthy aging, keeping you mentally sharp, emotionally grounded, and physically capable. In other words, resilience is your golden ticket to a life filled with joy, connection, and vitality.

A Resilient Mindset for Every Season

As life evolves, so will your resilience. The goals you set in your 50s might look different in your 70s or 80s, and that's okay. Resilience is about adaptability—knowing when to push and when to give yourself grace. It's about embracing each stage of life with curiosity and a sense of adventure. Did you once dream of running marathons but now prefer long, leisurely walks? That's resilience at work, shifting with your needs and keeping you moving forward. Resilience isn't about clinging to old expectations; it's about embracing new possibilities with open arms.

Aging With a Resilient Heart

Healthy aging is more than just staying physically fit. It's about cultivating a heart and mind that are open, curious, and resilient. Every small choice you make today—whether it's trying a new hobby, connecting with a friend, or simply pausing to take a deep breath—is an investment systematic review and meta- analysis. Ageing Research Reviews. 2022; 77: 101594.

45. Lee LO, Grodstein F, Trudel-Fitzgerald C, James P, Okuzono SS, Koga HK, et al. Optimism, Daily Stressors, and Emotional Well-Being Over Two Decades in a Cohort of Aging Men. J Gerontol B Psychol Sci Soc Sci. 2022; 77 (8): 1373-83.

Frailty And Nutrition: Powering Resilience

"Frailty and Nutrition: Powering Resilience" is a simple, useful guide that helps you face the challenges of aging with strength and energy. It explains how proper nutrition can boost resilience and fight frailty, focusing on the importance of key nutrients and gut health. With clear advice and practical tips, it shows how to make smart food choices to stay physically, mentally, and socially healthy. Whether you want to prevent frailty or manage it better, this book is a helpful tool for living a healthier, more independent life. Ideal for older adults, caregivers, and anyone who wants to age well.

Frailty And Fitness: The Transformative Power Of Exercise

Frailty often seems like an inevitable companion of aging, but it does not have to be. "Frailty and Fitness: The Transformative Power of Exercise" is your comprehensive guide to understanding this condition and reclaiming vitality through the power of movement. Packed with practical advice, this book delves into the science of frailty, revealing how targeted exercises can help rebuild strength, improve balance, and restore independence.

From resistance and power training to overcoming barriers and designing personalized programs, this book provides actionable steps for individuals at all levels of fitness. Discover inspiring stories, easy-to-follow exercises, and the latest research on how exercise not only combats physical frailty but also enhances mental and social well-being.

Whether you are an older adult looking to regain confidence or a caregiver aiming to support someone you love, "Frailty and Fitness: The Transformative Power of Exercise" offers the tools you need to embrace an active, healthy lifestyle. Start small, stay consistent, and watch how even modest efforts can lead to transformative results. Empower yourself to age with strength, resilience, and joy —because it is never too late to rewrite your story.

Frailty And Heart Health: Understanding The Relationship For A Healthier Future

Dive into the fascinating and crucial connection between frailty and heart health in this engaging and informative book. Written in a warm, approachable style, "Frailty and Heart Health" unravels the science behind these intertwined health challenges, exploring how they impact our bodies, minds, and daily lives as we age.

Discover sensible insights into the shared risk factors, warning signs, and biological pathways that link frailty and heart health. With easy-to-follow advice on nutrition, exercise, and medical care, this book empowers readers to take control of their health. From recognizing the first signs of frailty to navigating recovery after heart events, this is your guide to building resilience and thriving at every stage of life.

Whether you are a caregiver, a healthcare professional, or someone eager to age well, this book offers hope, knowledge, and tools to add not just years to your life, but life to your years.

(References included within the book for deeper exploration.)